Karolina Rzadkowolska

Euphoric

An Eight-Week Plan to Ditch Alcohol and Reclaim Your Life

PIATKUS

PIATKUS

First published in the United States in 2022 by Harper Horizon,
an imprint of HarperCollins Focus LLC
First published in Great Britain in 2022 by Piatkus

A CIP catalogue record for this book
is available from the British Library.

ISBN: 978-0-349-42938-0

Printed and bound in Great Britain by Clays Ltd, Elcograf S.p.A.

Papers used by Piatkus are from well-managed forests
and other responsible sources.

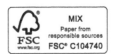

This book is written as a source of information about the effects of alcohol.
It is based on the research and observations of the author, who is not a medical
doctor. The information contained in this book should by no means be considered
a substitute for the advice of a qualified medical professional, who should always be
consulted before beginning any diet or other health program. The author and the
publisher expressly disclaim responsibility for any adverse effects arising from
the use or application of the information contained in this book.

Names and identifying characteristics of some individuals
have been changed to preserve their privacy.

Piatkus
An imprint of
Little, Brown Book Group
Carmelite House
50 Victoria Embankment
London EC4Y 0DZ

An Hachette UK Company
www.hachette.co.uk

www.littlebrown.co.uk

dla Babci

CONTENTS

CONTENTS

PART III
YOUR EIGHT-WEEK PLAN
TO DITCH ALCOHOL AND GAIN
A HAPPIER, MORE CONFIDENT YOU

Why You're Meant to Be Here

can't believe I love mornings so much. I used to sleep through all of this. I wake up right before the sunrise. My sleep was deep, uninterrupted, and I love remembering my dreams. After I have a brief dance party to fully wake up while my coffee brews, I grab my laptop and start writing. I love to write first thing in the morning when I'm most creative, then I do some gratitude journaling and goal setting. Afterward, I listen to a guided meditation instructing me to visualize my dream life. I visualize my dream day, down to what I do on a perfect morning. My visualization isn't far off from what I am doing right now.

I go on a run around my neighborhood. It's dewy outside, and the sun spotlights little patches of leaves—it feels like I'm witnessing a secret. I arrive home, stretch, and shower. By 8:00 a.m., I'm ready to start my workday.

Before I connect with my dream clients, I make an executive plan for the day. Every day I get to do what I love most—help women discover their best selves—all because I stopped playing small and living my life on other people's terms.

WHY GOING ALCOHOL-FREE WAS THE BEST DECISION OF MY LIFE

My life isn't perfect and offers plenty of learning opportunities. But I'm no longer hoping or wishing for my dream life. I'm building it every day.

Would you believe me if I told you this dream life all started with a decision to reevaluate the role of alcohol in my life? Just one short break from drinking was all it took to fall in love with my new life and way of being so much that I decided, *Why settle for hangovers and mediocrity ever again?* In fact, I am thrilled I don't have to drink anymore. I feel extremely lucky.

Not only do I feel better, look better, and sleep better, ditching alcohol has allowed me to hear my intuition loud and clear and pursue the bigger purpose of my life. Living alcohol-free has been the gateway to greater confidence, authentic friendships, and wholehearted self-love. After years of feeling stuck and unfulfilled, taking a break from alcohol ended up being the fastest road to my biggest dreams—dreams like becoming an author, running my own successful business, uplifting women all over the world and helping them believe in their greater dreams, traveling whenever I want, and being friends with my heroes. Being alcohol-free is a dream lifestyle. You could say I'm euphoric.

Maybe something in your mind is slamming on the brakes right now. Before we proceed, let's tackle the big, fat elephant in the room, the question you may be asking yourself:

Isn't giving up drinking a bit too extreme and only a thing for brown-paper-bag, sitting-on-a-park-bench types?

You see, that was my dominant thought for years. I assumed that the only reason you'd stop doing something unhealthy like drinking was because you had a massive problem. Not just because you might want to get, er, healthier. What a strange paradox! Think about it: If I were to quit or cut back on sugar or fast food, or start working out more, would anyone accuse me of having a problem? Yet, as a society, outdated thinking attaches so much stigma and shame around alcohol. And it keeps too many people stuck in a habit that ultimately isn't making them happy.

Take my life, for example. I had turned thirty years old and realized that thinking about alcohol consumed valuable mind space. I wasn't obsessing over where my next drink was or making sure I had enough alcohol at home—I was thinking about the dilemma, a constant tug-of-war in my mind of *should I or shouldn't I?* I constantly wanted to drink less yet couldn't figure it out. Not only that, but something was missing and felt off in my life. As though I was wasting my gifts and potential on something irrelevant—a *beverage*. While I could brush these thoughts away as I was planning my next wine country getaway, I heard them loud and clear in the still and quiet mornings. I knew it when I again woke up with a dull headache. I knew it when I let myself down and broke a self-imposed rule (no more than two drinks) and felt my self-esteem crumbling. I knew it when I journaled that, surely, I was meant for more than this merry-go-round of being good, healthy, and productive all week, only to overdrink on the weekend and nullify all my efforts.

Yet it was hard for me to articulate all of this as a problem. I didn't drink out of sadness. I didn't drink every day. It was a social thing or a weekend treat. Sushi nights, dinner parties, game nights, and of course, Netflix and wine on Saturday and Sunday to unwind. While it all looked normal, I had many rules, trying so damn hard to find the elusive balance. I couldn't for the life of me figure out why alcohol was my

Achilles' heel. Of course, I felt shitty when I overdid it. But I also felt lousy after one or two. What was I doing wrong, and why couldn't I make alcohol work in my life? Each Monday, I resolved to play around with the equation. No strong beers. No more than two drinks. No drinking before 7:00 p.m.

After years of this internal turbulence, I finally decided to take a break: Dry January, a popular time to take a month-long break from alcohol. It gave me the excuse I needed to try life without alcohol and avoid having to go around and ring everyone to say I had a problem. I saw it as a way to reset and internalize new, mindful drinking habits. I never expected it to turn me on to life so much that I eventually couldn't settle for rough sleep and booze breath ever again. My alcohol-free month was amazing. I slept well, lived my ideal healthy lifestyle, devoured books, and felt a shift in my appreciation and gratitude. I enjoyed myself while doing the simplest things, like playing board games with my husband, Robert, and goofing around with my niece. I learned that I could hang out with my closest friends without drinking and still have fun. I felt like myself—no masks, no internal shame smothering me, just me learning to be awake and alive.

Come February, I wasn't looking forward to drinking again. But I didn't think I had a choice. Have you ever gone on a vacation and realized that life is short, and you should do what makes you happiest? Then you return home, wake up on Monday morning, and slog through a job you hate? That's how it felt. Just like I didn't see any alternatives outside the nine-to-five rut, I believed normal adults had to drink.

I drank again that February—nine times—and I hated each and every time with a heightened awareness. It was the little things that ticked me off. Drinking stole away my nightly routine. Hard to read and journal when you're buzzed. I hated how I felt in the morning after ridiculously restless sleep compared to the sleeping-beauty slumber I'd grown accustomed to during my break. I noticed how upbeat, energetic, and appreciative I was while not drinking. Only one drink in, I'd turn apathetic, impatient, and easily frustrated, even starting fights with my husband. Drinking sucked.

That was the moment I decided to take another break. Except when I got to the end of this next thirty days, magical things happened. I was riding a pink cloud, a burst of happiness. I felt giddy, like I was falling in love. Thirty days turned into sixty days. I traveled to New Orleans, Hawaii, and Japan, all while alcohol-free. I watched sunrises. I swam in crystal-clear waters and rode bikes along the coast. I felt thunderstruck by thousand-year-old temples. I went to birthday parties and dinner parties and enjoyed a new sense of poise and grace. I felt lucky that I wasn't going to wake up feeling unwell, compared to anyone drinking around me. I was growing and also writing voraciously. It's been my lifelong dream to write, but I used to have the worst writer's block. And when I took all of this and evaluated whether this new path was worth pursuing, compared to a beer I've had like three thousand times before, all I could say was "been there, done that." This life was too good to give up.

With that, I started chasing the woman I was meant to be. I got crystal clear on what my biggest dreams were, and instead of feeling stuck and afraid, I went after them. One baby step after another, I built my Euphoric Alcohol-Free business, became a certified alcohol-free life coach, launched *Euphoric the Podcast*, ran a half-marathon, left my day job, spoke publicly about how amazing life is without drinking, and wrote a book (this one!). Today, I do what I love most in the world and help women experience the same transformation and incredible shifts in their lives, by changing their relationship with alcohol. I've worked with thousands of soulful women (and men) who want more out of life than hangovers and are ready to completely reinvent themselves. Feeling just as stuck as I was, this one change triggers an avalanche of transformation in their lives, ultimately leading them to clarity on their greater purpose and their dreams. At the end of the day, it's not about a beverage—it's about being awake to your life!

I'll show you how to do the same, because you deserve to have this eye-opening experience and evaluate for yourself which lifestyle you prefer. Which one is more aligned with your values? Which one empowers you to pursue your bigger dreams? Which one allows you to believe that anything is possible for you and that you're done playing small on the sidelines?

But before we begin, let's clear up some assumptions and misinformation about alcohol use, which might be holding you back.

THE NEW, UNHEALTHY NORMAL

Most of us have an idea of what problem drinking looks like, from examples in movies, books, or our lives. The woman who picks up her kids from school with vodka in her tumbler. The homeless man drinking on the side of the road. The friend who was utterly consumed by alcohol, hit rock bottom, and now spends the rest of her days attending Alcoholics Anonymous (AA) meetings. In our minds, this is what problem drinking looks like, and to establish a category that is *not* that, we use the term "normal drinker." Normal drinkers have their life together, drink routinely but not overwhelmingly, and all in all are doing okay. The thing is, our definition of normal drinking is constantly expanding to new, unhealthy standards. Most drinkers are overdrinking, and it's called "normal" because it's become the normative behavior in our society.

The drinking guidelines made by health and medical associations are strict. No more than one drink per occasion. Maybe two for a male, though it depends what country you live in (countries like the United Kingdom are tightening these standards to match the latest recommendations in health research).[1] And the definition of a drink is far less than what we're being served. A pint of craft beer at 7 percent alcohol is way above the standard of 350ml of 5 percent beer. A restaurant pour of 175ml of a heavy cabernet (at 15 percent alcohol) is much more than the standard of 150ml of 12 percent wine.[2] If one drink is the acceptable, healthy standard, how many people regularly drink more than that? How about almost every drinker I know? Does that mean we're all alcoholics? No. Drinking isn't binary like that. It's on a huge spectrum of different norms, consumption levels, and behaviors. The Centers for Disease Control and Prevention finds that most people who overdrink aren't alcoholics or alcohol dependent.[3] Those of us who find ourselves in between light, occasional drinking and all-day-every-day drinking are in the majority.

According to the Substance Abuse and Mental Health Administration, 59 percent of regular drinkers misuse alcohol and drink way more than the health guidelines recommend.[4] Yes, most drinkers! Meaning that overdrinking is the norm. No one bats an eye at bottomless brunch. Or dinner parties with free-flowing wine. Or a day of beer tasting. And when you think about it, it's all around you. Do your friends stop at one drink? Are you the only person you know who drinks every week? Hardly. When you see it all around you, it's easy to internalize the idea that drinking like this isn't that bad for you.

A whole bottle of vodka? Bad. A few glasses of wine after work? No problem.

Not only is this the new normal but drinking per the health guidelines seems like a singularity. The Centers for Disease Control also says that two drinks a day for a woman is considered heavy drinking.[5] What?! If I had limited myself to two drinks on a Friday night out with my friends, I would have thought I was the healthiest person around! Yet studies show that alcohol consumption in the last two decades is on the rise, especially among women.[6] When you're a routine drinker, you likely have a bit of "complicated" thrown into your relationship with alcohol. Studies show that 52 percent of Americans are trying to drink less.[7] It's not because they're saints. They want to drink less because they aren't happy with the way alcohol is showing up in their life. Welcome to the silent majority.

While this situation might not be *that* bad, it's also not letting you live life to its fullest. This murky middle ground often feels like living life on a merry-go-round. You wake up on a Monday morning after drinking, feeling out of it, and resolve to do better. The week is spent doing good things: drinking green juice, going to yoga classes, eating well, and meditating. Then, like a toxic boyfriend, alcohol shows up and throws you in a tailspin of unhealthy patterns and poor decisions. Detox just to retox, feeling crazy on this never-ending loop.

But many of us fear that if we even start to examine our relationship with alcohol, we'll automatically be labeled as someone who has a "problem" with alcohol. And who wants that? So we sweep it all under a rug—the tiredness, the "hangxiety," the guilt, the shame—and pretend everything is fine. Meanwhile, deep down, we believe something is inherently wrong with us because we can't figure out the right balance of alcohol in our lives. And because alcohol can be a taboo topic, we get no assurance that this is a common problem and can feel lonely and isolated.

One of my clients came to me thinking something must be wrong with her. She didn't drink large amounts, yet her body wasn't tolerating it. She believed her body was worse at processing alcohol than other people's and had no idea that everyone gets worse at processing alcohol over time.

Alcohol is the only drug we have to defend not partaking in. It's pushed on some of us as early as our teen years and is a constant presence in our culture when we celebrate, socialize, relax, and commiserate. Combine societal conditioning, the science of habit formation, and an addictive substance, and it's no wonder many of us have complicated relationships with alcohol. And the only way we've been taught to deal with the matter is to ascertain whether we have a drinking problem with a capital P.

Trying to figure out if my drinking was normal or abnormal was an enigma. I partied hard in college and grad school and had nonexistent coping mechanisms save drinking, but as I got older, I made a lot of changes to tone it down and get healthier. By the time I was thirty, I considered myself both a healthy and mindful person. Sometimes I moderated; sometimes I didn't. Sometimes I'd feel highly virtuous for having only one or two drinks. Other times I'd feel extreme shame for having a zillion at a party. I tried hard to be disciplined, to keep it all balanced, and to make strict rules for myself and my drinking. But the thing is, I never knew which Karolina would come out on any given night, the poised graceful one or the one who overdrank. When the wrong one did and I drank too much, I felt like someone had hijacked my body and brain. Yet I didn't drink most days, I had no issue with alcohol in my house, and I drank less year after year. Was I normal or an alcoholic? How about normal-ish?

Trying to figure out whether you're "normal" or have a problem is like trying to figure out how much longer you should work at a job you hate, even though it makes you sick and tired, because you get good health benefits. It doesn't matter if you have a problem or not, or what terms you use to label or justify your drinking. The question you need to ask is: *Does it make me happy?*

Is my drinking habit aligned with my values? Does it let me feel exceptional joy, retain my integrity, feel 100 percent, and show up for the ones I love? Does it serve me in chasing my wildest dreams? A complicated relationship with alcohol comes with a lot of internal conflict that takes up space in your mental landscape—space that could be used to live out your fullest potential. You don't have to have a drinking problem for alcohol to be holding you back from your most radiant self.

SOBER CURIOUS?

I'm so happy that you're here. Together, we're going to start a wellness revolution. Your curiosity about a new way of being is the gateway to huge shifts in your life, to feeling euphoric, passionate, and alive with purpose. You're part of a growing trend of people who value health and consciousness. You don't take societal norms at face value. You're here, ready to question your relationship with alcohol, and through this journey, experience the greatest personal growth exercise of your life. You're brave enough to question your drinking habits and realize your curiosity is empowering, not embarrassing. You're ready to challenge yourself to take a break and see if alcohol truly does allow you to live your best life. Then, with that information, you choose whether you want to go back or not. Spoiler alert: research by One Year No Beer found that 87 percent of people who take an extended break from alcohol don't go back to drinking.[8] What they discover on the other side is so good, they're forever changed.

Take Elena. While partying was her thing when she was younger, as a mom in her midthirties, her life is filled with organic foods, no-waste practices, and a conscious approach to life and parenthood. When she took a break from alcohol, everything clicked into place. The mindful, healthy, and meaningful lifestyle she desired was found in alcohol-free living. While she worked hard to set boundaries around her drinking, she realized she didn't have to drink a lot to feel that alcohol was holding her back, not to mention making her groggy the following mornings. What she discovered on the other side was inner peace, freedom, and a life fully aligned with her values. She felt a natural high, daily inspiration to try new things, and a waterfall of creativity for her business.

Most of my clients are incredibly healthy and mindful women. In fact, drinking is often the one incongruency in their otherwise holistic lifestyle. This kind of incongruence is incredibly painful and a huge source of internal conflict. Psychologists call this *cognitive dissonance*, meaning that you believe two opposing thoughts at the same time.[9] Like when your higher self tells you to consume less alcohol or none at all, yet something inside you tells you to pour a drink at 6:00 p.m. Or when you call yourself a healthy person yet wake up feeling physically unwell after a night of drinking. In this book, I'll share the mindset shifts you need to get the memo to your subconscious and fully align with your values and dispel the cognitive dissonance.

And you don't need to feel deprived, experience FOMO (fear of missing out), or worry that your social life will take a nosedive, because I'm going to teach you how to take an eight-week break from alcohol the right way. Working on changing your habits is great, but doing so leaves a deprivation vacuum if you don't change your mindset. I'll teach you to love being alcohol-free the same way someone loves being vegetarian. Do you think vegetarians bemoan to themselves that they can't eat meat? Go around missing it? Throw themselves a pity party? Or do they love their choices, knowing they hold the secret to longevity and an ethical lifestyle, convinced that they know something the rest of us don't?

Alcohol is a sleep-interrupting, cancer-causing, brain-altering, depression-producing, fulfillment-robbing, confidence-faking substance that quashes your natural drive. Soon enough, you'll be thrilled that you don't have to drink it anymore.

And here's what you can expect from me during our time together: In parts I and II, I'll show you why you should take a break from alcohol. We'll review the health benefits and personal-growth epiphanies (from body, mind, and soul). My hope is that this kind of life will look so expansive, so ripe with possibility, that trying an alcohol-free challenge will seem like a no-brainer. In part III, I'll show you how to live alcohol-free with my eight-week plan, which is modeled after my most successful course, Become Euphoric™, and my coaching framework. Not only will you discover insights about yourself and change your entire thinking about drinking, you will be on a path to uplevel your life and stop settling for mediocrity in any part of it.

If you want more support and celebrations during your

breakthroughs, join the Euphoric community. I even have some bonus goodies, just for you, that will make this journey even more fun, at www.euphoricaf.com/book-bonus.

I fully believe that all people, no matter their drinking habits, can try another way without being judged or stigmatized. You're allowed to explore alcohol-free living if . . .

- You hate how you feel after a night out.
- You're not sure whether your daily wine with dinner is serving you.
- Drinking makes you feel unmotivated the next day.
- You find it hard and stressful to moderate.
- You want to sleep better, lose weight, or be a better role model for your children.
- Your intuition tells you this is the key to achieving your bigger dreams.

Every reason under the sun is valid for you to be here, to reevaluate an outdated relationship with alcohol or unconscious habit. Alcohol-free is the next wellness revolution, and no one needs to adopt a label to try it.

ARE YOU READY?

Remember this: Change is never easy. Getting out of your comfort zone is hard, and drinking happens to be an ultimate comfort-zone behavior. The part of you that doesn't want to change will scream at you with excuses and limiting stories about what this means for your life. But I know you've done hard things before and felt wildly fulfilled afterward. And I know you've also taken it easy and felt stuck and regretful. Ever heard the saying that everything you want in life is outside your comfort zone? If you have an inkling, however tiny, that alcohol is holding you back from your dream life, you deserve to explore that inner wisdom to its fullest. I promise you—you won't regret it. It will open the door to more self-love, confidence, and a purpose-driven life.

If you're ready to experience life fully alive, keep reading!

PART I

Your Body

CHAPTER 1

Going Alcohol-Free Is Like a Yoga Retreat

used to be captivated by Buddhist monks. I'd picture a monk sitting peacefully on a deck overlooking a serene body of water and think, *I wish that could be me.* I yearned for such an existence and believed that if I could have what the monk had, I'd have peace of mind and freedom from my drama. In my little fantasy, there was no alcohol, and no matter what, the monk woke up every morning rested and calm. He lived a simple lifestyle with meaningful rituals and long stretches of deep contemplation. His moods weren't an up-and-down roller coaster. Instead, he experienced stillness, and love in his heart.

Have you ever yearned for such an existence? Perhaps you've never considered monkhood, but I bet spiritual well-being is high on your wellness wish list. Maybe a yoga retreat would be your thing. If I stumbled on an unexpected few thousand dollars, I'd spend it on a yoga retreat on some distant tropical island. It sounds like the ultimate bliss: eating vegan food, doing active and restorative exercise, and having no distractions or places to go other than inside my mind. Taking care of myself in a primal and soothing way and healing my overactive brain.

Sound appealing to you too? If so, I have good news: going alcohol-free is like stepping through the resort villa doors. First off, alcohol-free living dramatically enhances your well-being. In part I, I'll share with you how everything, from your sleep to your brain chemistry, rebalances and improves, leaving you not only feeling healthier but also much happier. This is the ultimate healing exercise that makes you feel better. And since alcohol ultimately numbs your thoughts, feelings, and emotions, the extended break gives you a chance to be introspective and to know yourself in a new way. You'll become more present and aware of your inner desires and needs, as I'll share in part II. This is a journey to know yourself more fully and love yourself more deeply. When the present version of you does things with the future version of you in mind, you'll feel more loved and cared for.

And let's not forget about the epiphanies you'll have. This retreat is also about determining what you want in life and giving you the drive, confidence, and motivation to go after it. In part III, you'll apply everything you've learned to your life—by taking an eight-week break from alcohol—and focus on your bigger why. My favorite part of doing this work is seeing women's dreams flutter back to them, as well as their determination to make them happen. Those someday goals that have been sitting on the back burner? With the mental energy, time, and drive you reclaim, suddenly *someday* won't be good enough, and you'll want to work on those goals today.

Keep in mind that taking a break will have challenges. A yoga retreat isn't easy either. You're not even allowed to use your phone! When things get hard, you can't escape to watch TV. You can't eat away your feelings with a pint of Ben & Jerry's.

A yoga retreat puts you front and center with your emotions and feelings, and you can't duck them with escapist tendencies that bring you straight back to your comfort zone. Taking a break from alcohol might feel hard at times, because you allow yourself to feel everything, even the uncomfortable and the painful. Remember that quick fixes never work, and your emotions are meant to be processed and learned from. This journey will grow your emotional capacity and resiliency, teach you to cope in much healthier ways, and help you come out on the other side with freedom, mental peace, and a hunger to design your dream life. This is the ultimate personal growth and wellness exercise, and the rewards will far outweigh the discomfort.

WHY YOUR BODY WILL LOVE YOU

You already may have recognized this intuitively, but let me spell it out loud and clear: the aftereffects of drinking get much worse in your thirties and forties. By the time I was in my late twenties, my ability to bounce back from a night of drinking vanished, and even a few drinks did me in, resulting in rough sleep and waking up on the wrong side of the bed. Women come to me with this dilemma all the time and don't understand why even a few glasses of wine, which was no problem in their twenties, set them so far back the next day. And if you drink almost every day, this tiredness might be normal for you. You might even assume that's just what it feels like to get older.

I've had women disappointedly share with me that something must be wrong with their bodies, for them to not be able to process alcohol well anymore. However, nothing is wrong with their bodies—or with yours. In fact, it's trying to tell you exactly what it wants and needs. There's a reason it's easier to pull an all-nighter when you're eighteen than when you're forty. Your body doesn't want you to do it! With alcohol, your body is giving you the exact same signals.

Alcohol, or ethanol, is a toxic substance that takes a lot of effort for your body to detoxify from. While trace amounts of alcohol are found in certain products, like bread, kombucha, and even fruit, the most comprehensive studies have deemed the amount we ingest in alcoholic drinks is unsafe. The ethanol in your drink is the same ethanol used to fuel cars and rockets and found in your house paint and used as a chemical solvent in the heaviest of industries. It's the same ethanol in your hand sanitizer, used to kill living organisms. I won't detail every awful health effect here, but if you've ever gone on any diet to improve how you feel, eliminating alcohol would probably make the biggest difference. Just think about how many options we have today: vegetarian, caffeine-free, dairy-free, sugar-free, gluten-free, vegan, paleo, and so on. With so many socially acceptable lifestyles that involve giving up entire substances or food groups, is it really so crazy to go alcohol-free? Must there be a "story" behind why you're alcohol-free or a stigma in choosing not to drink?

As a substance that not only affects your physical body but also heightens your anxiety and lowers your mood, taking a break is a self-care must. You deserve to see what your body feels like in its natural state. To feel fully alive and energetic. To know the freedom that comes with removing your desires to drink. To be free of unconscious habits and cultural norms. To experience the full breadth of life and awaken to your natural drive. To love yourself so much you don't even want to drink.

Let's start by focusing on the physical benefits, and you'll learn why your body is going to love you. To experience true wellness and introspection, let's hop off the merry-go-round of volatile emotions, tiredness, and doing things just to fit in. The next few chapters will explore these changes in your mood, energy, and well-being, and the direct results you can expect. Get ready to be happier, more energetic, and better rested than you've ever been.

CHAPTER 2

Create Mornings that You Love

NO MORE HANGOVERS!

It's an obvious benefit that can't be overstated: When you don't drink, you're never hungover. Ever. Can you imagine waking up almost every single morning feeling amazing? Even at 5:00 or 6:00 a.m.? It's incredible. The word *hangover* might be charged, but if I drank the night before, even a glass or two, I definitely felt the worse for wear. And, of course, sometimes I was really sick. I'd attend a party or some kind of drinking festival and wake up the next morning with a debilitating headache. Lucky me if it was Saturday or Sunday and I could stay in bed most of the day. If not, I counted the hours until I could get back to bed. I was physically sick and tried hard to sleep it off.

As I got older, much less alcohol put me in this state. I felt a hint of this grossness every time after I drank. Even one drink ruined my sleep and made me tired the next day. How about a couple glasses of wine after not drinking all week? The next day, I'd have the heaviest headache, where my brain felt like it was being squeezed. Handful of beers on a Friday night? Saturday morning I'd feel *fuzzy*.

It's a life-changer to wake up feeling great, and I want that for you! Waking up at 6:00 a.m. is my new high. How you wake up sets the tone for the rest of the day. When I woke up with a headache or felt *bleh*, I couldn't be bothered that day. I'd get fast food, watch a ton of TV, and phone it in. When you don't drink, you wake up feeling more upbeat because your body isn't working overtime to detox even a little from the night before.

Be patient, because the first few days off may not be a picnic, especially if you're used to drinking often. Some people report feeling weary, getting headaches, and having trouble sleeping. It can take one to three weeks for the body to completely detoxify itself and recalibrate.[1] (Quick but important side note: If you have a physical addiction to alcohol, please seek medical attention, because alcohol withdrawal can be dangerous. I am not a doctor, and my experiences and those of my clients do not represent severe alcohol use disorder.)

But trust me, things only get better. Your body repairs and rebalances, and you'll feel more rested and energetic. And soon enough, it'll be hard to imagine you ever voluntarily made yourself feel ill or not 100 percent your best. My client Lisa tells me that waking up hangover-free is "like a gift I give myself every single day."

Every weekend, the alcohol-free community on Instagram celebrates being hangover-free. It doesn't get old. And it's a big deal! How you wake up each morning defines how you live your day, and how your live your days defines how you live your life.

I mean, can we talk about how gross it feels to wake up after a night of drinking? Because it doesn't seem like society does. Alcohol is all things rosy and fun, and we gloss over the fact that it also makes you feel grosser than a beached whale.

Like the dreary sleep you fall in and out of all morning, hoping that the next time you open your eyes, you'll feel better. How about waking up and burping hoppy beer or wine tannins? So gross you could throw up right then and there. Sweating in my bed (yes, I've been there and so have you), my mouth reeking, gagging from reflux, my stomach on fire from acid. Disgusting and depressing at the same time. The horror, the horror we've regularly put ourselves through! And if I experienced these effects after three or so drinks, I think it's safe to assume this grossness is happening to most people too.

Don't we drink because it's supposed to make us feel good? But a few spikes of dopamine manipulation each week, followed by incredible lows, is nothing compared to the joy and well-being that you can feel *all the time* when you're alcohol-free. When you embark on your challenge, each morning you'll want to take a moment to express gratitude for the wellness you get to feel every day. And appreciate how much better your sleep is. Because the effects of alcohol on sleep are huge.

THE SLEEPING BEAUTY SLEEP

Alcohol and poor-quality sleep are deeply intertwined. I had enough experience with drinking nights versus nondrinking nights to know that my nondrinking sleep was like floating gently among the clouds compared to my postdrinking sleep, which was like finding myself in a rowboat at sea in the middle of a hurricane. I'd toss and turn, sweat, and feel my body was stressed all night, like it was fighting a war.

I had no idea what was going on and why alcohol was preventing restful sleep. I think I was twenty-five when I realized even one glass of wine disrupted my beauty rest. And by the time I ditched drinking for good, I wasn't young and dumb anymore. I couldn't ignore the effects or bounce back like an eighteen-year-old.

For someone who purposely ruined my sleep, I was obsessed with it. I always tried to get more because I was perpetually exhausted. If I drank, I tried to go to bed early or sleep in, so I could attempt to sleep off the alcohol. If I had two or three glasses of wine, I required the perfect sleeping conditions—a fan, a mask, a special pillow, and no early wake-up noises—or else I was dooming an already bad situation to be even worse. Did you ever drink the night before, expecting to sleep in, and then get woken up by someone else? Oh boy, did this make me angry. Or how about feeling unwell on a workday or a day filled with tons of to-dos? So wretched.

But the absolute worst were the 4:00 a.m. wake-ups. Your eyes pop open, your heart races, you feel a knot in the pit of your stomach, and you slowly realize: you did it to yourself again. You drank more than you wanted to. Not much is worse than the doom and gloom of the 4:00 a.m. wake-up. Everything wrong in your life is horribly apparent, you can't fall back asleep, and you tell yourself you'll never put yourself through this ever again. Even that feels like a lie though, because you've already been in this position so many times. My 4:00 a.m. wake-ups were depressing and anxiety-ridden. And the horrible thing was that I thought they were my problem alone. That no one else could possibly be going through this, otherwise, wouldn't I have heard about it? The situation was soul-crushing and isolating, and I thought something was uniquely wrong with me.

But it wasn't. What I was going through, what you've been going through—the rough sleep, the 4:00 a.m. wake-ups—is normal when you consume alcohol. When I share with a client how common this is, the response is often a sigh of relief. Anyone who drinks has experienced something like this. It's crazy how much we assume something is wrong with us, instead of rightly blaming the drink. All this drama I describe above is the effect of alcohol on the human body.

Alcohol is a depressant and slows down your central nervous system. It eventually induces sleep, and many people believe that a drink helps them get to bed—20 percent of Americans misguidedly use alcohol to help them fall asleep.[2] While alcohol does help with sleep onset, it's ineffective for deep rest, and the only reason it helps you fall asleep is because it's sedating you into slow-wave sleep for the first half of the night.

Slow-wave sleep is considered a downstate, in which your neurons are silent and resting. It's important for the rebuilding and repairing of muscles and tissues. It seems deep and solid, and usually isn't accompanied by dreaming. Normally, we cycle between slow-wave sleep and rapid-eye movement (REM) sleep in ninety-minute cycles throughout the night, needing about five or so cycles to feel rested. However, drinking alcohol throws off that balance, and studies show that, after drinking, people spend the first half of the night in deep slow-wave sleep and less time in REM sleep.[3] It might feel deep, but we're skipping the important REM sleep, and the body is working hard to metabolize the alcohol. Anyway, we know from experience that any deep sleep is short-lived, and the second half of the night is fragmented.

Remember when I said alcohol is a depressant? As the body metabolizes alcohol, the sedative effects wear off about five hours after your last drink,[4] quite possibly waking you up at a crisp 3:00 or 4:00 in the morning, thirsty and restless. But there's more to it. Our bodies are constantly trying to achieve homeostasis, even when we guzzle, eat, and breathe in toxins.

To counter a depressant like alcohol, our bodies release stress hormones and neuropeptides, like cortisol, adrenaline, dynorphin, and corticotropin-releasing factor.[5] While you might not have heard of dynorphin, think of it as the opposite of endorphins—it makes you feel sad. Combined, these stimulants make you feel anxious, low, wired, and exhausted. And you'll feel them the most about five hours after drinking.

After drinking, I usually went to bed at 11:00 p.m. and had my startled wake-up at 4:00 a.m.—five round hours after drinking. Of course my body felt like it had just been shot full of adrenaline—it really was! It would be so hard to fall back asleep. And my mind raced with heart-wrenching anxiety over what I'd said or done or how I'd broken a promise to myself, yet again. The rest of the early morning hours would be spent with frequent awakenings and light sleep. To top it off, the stress hormones circulate in your body for much longer, leaving you feeling stressed, anxious, and gloomy the next day (or days). Thanks, alcohol. Studies even prove that as you continue drinking over time, your body releases more stress hormones.[6] Maybe that's why we could all roll with the punches in college but have no stomach for it after the age of twenty-five.

Okay, okay—so all I needed to do is drink less, right? After all, my 4:00 a.m. wake-ups didn't happen every night, just the nights when I drank too much (and by "too much," let's say three-plus drinks). Maybe I should have kept it under two drinks? Unfortunately, studies show that all dosages of alcohol increase sleep disruption during the second half of the night and decrease total REM sleep.[7] REM sleep is what's known as dreaming sleep and was first discovered when observers noticed fast eye movement during sleep experiments. It's vital for brain nourishment and helps process memories from short term to long term. It also helps process our emotions, especially negative ones, while we dream. Negative dreams are important, because they can help us better experience our emotions and build more resilience in our waking life.[8] As I mentioned before, the average human spends the night in five sleep cycles, each culminating in REM sleep and lasting about ninety minutes per cycle.

You may be in bed all night, but you could be getting as little as one or two REM cycles when you drink, effectively robbing you of the sleep your brain needs to process and develop. Even if you clock in eight hours after a night of drinking, you aren't getting the nourishing sleep your body needs and will wake up feeling tired. Quality sleep is equally important as, if not more important than, the quantity. Alcohol's effect on sleep is so well-known it's standard for sleep advocates and health magazines to recommend avoiding alcohol before bed.

Lack of quality sleep has been linked to a host of health issues and is directly tied to life expectancy. It can make you feel lethargic, cranky, sad, and short-tempered, and can lead to cancer, diabetes, and depression. And one night's bad sleep can hardly be made up for on other nights. Studies show that it takes four days for your body to recapture just one hour of lost sleep.[9] So if you overstress your body every weekend but take it easy during the week, you'll never capture this lost sleep. Some regular drinkers drink every day, but almost all regular drinkers drink every weekend (otherwise they wouldn't be regular drinkers, but occasional ones). This means most drinkers never give themselves enough time away from alcohol to regain the sleep they're always losing.

However, taking a break will rebalance your sleep patterns and invite in the most nourishing, yummy sleep you've ever had as an adult. I sleep so well. It hardly ever takes longer than five minutes for me to fall asleep, I rarely wake up in the middle of the night (which was unheard of in my drinking days), I remember my dreams, and I naturally wake up around 6:00 a.m. Sober sleep is one of the most luxurious delights. While it might take a bit for your sleep patterns to rebalance, most of my clients see a measured improvement within a matter of weeks, and they love to tell me when they've turned the corner into much better sleep. After a few weeks of healing, Mary told me, "My sleep is so heavenly!" Karen said that only a few days in she was "sleeping so much better." In addition to better-quality sleep, women in my community are also amazed to discover their new favorite time of day—the morning!

PEACEFUL AND PRODUCTIVE MORNINGS

The birds are chirping, dawn is cresting over the tree line, and it's beautifully quiet. I'm writing these words at 6:00 a.m., as the sky turns pink. Let's just say that when I was drinking, 6:00 a.m. was the worst time of the day. Are you a morning person? I wasn't—not since I became an adult (and a drinker) did I ever enjoy waking up before 9:00 a.m. For years, I had to be at work by 8:30 and would get out of bed at the last moment possible. On the weekend, I slept in until 9:00 a.m. Sometimes even later, depending on the night I'd had.

I'm guessing that some of your mornings are just plain rough, some are extremely sleepy, and most are spent valiantly wishing you could sleep more. But when you take your break, your morning experience will completely change. You'll wake up feeling glorious. Mornings will take on a whole new meaning. When your body and brain are no longer sleep deprived, you won't feel so tired, and you don't need as much sleep to feel rested. I used to try to clock more than eight hours of sleep, because I knew I needed it to sleep off the alcohol or catch up after a rough night. These days, I'm perfectly rested after a solid seven or eight hours.

With this fresh outlook on the start of the day, you might find yourself waking up earlier and doing something you love during your newfound time. My client Linda says mornings are now her favorite time of day. She gets up early and has the house to herself before her daughter wakes up. It's peaceful and gives her the time and space to design her day with intention. Having a morning routine like this changed my life as well.

Since I wasn't hungover, worse for wear, or sleep deprived, I asked myself, *Why not wake up earlier and try a morning routine?* The book that got me started was *The Miracle Morning* by Hal Elrod. Elrod presents the idea of waking up an hour or so earlier than needed, so you can work on your personal development. He recommends multiple activities, including meditating, journaling, saying affirmations, visualizing your dream life, reading, and exercising. It's a jam-packed hour! I knew I wanted to devote more time to writing every day, so I added writing to the mix and set my alarm for 5:45 a.m. The first week was hard and gloomy, but soon enough, I looked forward to my private, quiet hour spent working on me, before the chaos of the day started. I got to think, dream, create, and ground myself in my highest intentions. Today, my morning routine varies depending on what I'm focusing on, but it usually consists of writing, meditating, goal-setting, giving gratitude, and planning my day.

Do you find it hard to get out of bed in the morning? Sure, some mornings I'd rather stay cozy and sleep longer. But I feel so much better after my morning routine that this convinces me to get up and do it, knowing that while some mornings I may not "feel" like it, it's worth it. My client Becky, a busy mom of three, created a new ritual in her life: morning is not only her time away from parenting—it's when she focuses on her personal growth and passion projects. In week six of your eight-week plan, we'll craft a morning routine you love, and I'll give you my best tips to get your butt out of bed.

Morning is my favorite time of day. I love that first cup of coffee, how fresh everything feels, and my superwoman ability to get things done. I'm convinced your relationship to morning is bound to improve too. Instead of not being able to sleep in or sleep it off, you can reframe your morning. It's your hour, just for you. And when you find something you love doing that excites you—whether taking a walk outside, doing sun salutations with the sunrise, or writing your book, or some combination of activities—the way you think about mornings will transform.

The thing about a healthy and fulfilling morning is that it switches your me-time from late night to dawn. When you go-go-go all day, especially with kids in the house, late night is often the only time you can breathe and just be with yourself. But this time is usually accompanied by wine and Netflix. That late-night time can feel precious, but now you know how much that wine is robbing you of good-quality rest. You'll be thankful you went to bed and then woke up early, before anyone else, for some soulful me-time instead of watching reruns.

THE CULTURE IS SHIFTING

Over the weekend, I was walking by my old stomping grounds in Pacific Beach, a youngster party neighborhood in San Diego. I walked past a gastropub and noticed that all the patio umbrellas were branded Athletic Brewing. In fact, Athletic Brewing had opened a tasting room near me. Why am I telling you this? This company only makes nonalcoholic, craft beer. Imagine if, ten years ago, it was totally normal to order a craft, nonalcoholic beer when I went out with my friends. Imagine all the heartache I could have avoided.

The culture of what we drink is shifting. Young millennials and Gen Zers are drinking less than previous generations.[10] And new beverage companies are sprouting up left and right to show us that a night out doesn't need to come with a side of hangovers. Just because you're not drinking alcohol doesn't mean you have to live in a state of deprivation. Fancy a coffee cream stout or double IPA? Peanut butter stout or milkshake IPA? (Quite possibly the best beer I've ever had—thanks, Surreal Brewing!) Not only do all these drinks exist, they also don't give you a crazy headache the next day.

Adult botanical blends like Seedlip and Borrago can create the perfect cucumber gimlet or tonic. Alcohol-free spirits like Lyre's and Ritual can make any drink you want, from an old-fashioned to a whiskey sour. You can even buy premade, zero-proof cocktails like Curious Elixirs (their number two, a pineapple and ginger sensation) or Kin Euphorics, made with adaptogens and nootropics. Kin makes a nighttime blend with melatonin to help you sleep, and a daytime blend with a bit of caffeine and ginseng for a kick. Non-alcoholic wine is catching up too. Gruvi makes a lovely prosecco, and Ariel has some great reds.

Even alcohol companies are betting on the rise of alcohol-free drinks and investing crazy amount of money in these companies. A Morning Consult poll revealed that 46 percent of adults have purchased a nonalcoholic beer or cocktail.[11] It's a growing industry. You can go out and socialize, have an adult beverage, and live a healthy lifestyle without feeling lousy the next day.

Finding these alternative drinks early in my journey made me feel confident in my new lifestyle. I didn't have to worry as much about completely changing the habit—it's perfectly okay to decompress, socialize, or celebrate over drinks. Just change the drink. When you drink to have a treat or feel pampered, tap water won't cut it. Particularly when people are drinking seemingly special drinks around you, you don't want to feel left out. So don't! With all these new options, you can bring your own mocktail—BYOM.

It's not just nonalcoholic beverage companies that are on the rise. Mocktail bars and pop-ups are in cities around the world. The hippest establishments have mocktail menus. Even super-chefy restaurants are offering alcohol-free pairings with their ten-course tasting menus. Sober raves and dance parties are totally a thing, and these shifts prompt an important question: Why should the alcohol industry dominate nightlife? The alcohol-free life is a creative space with new options and fun possibilities. Why not get crafty in your kitchen and whip up a fun mocktail? I'll share with you my favorite homemade and easy-to-make recipes in the eight-week plan. The worst thing you could do is equate the alcohol-free life with deprivation. And there's no reason to do so, with all the fun and crafty alcohol-free drinks you can try.

CHAPTER 3

Feel Fully Alive

No more hangovers—check. Deep restful sleep every night—check. Beautiful mornings spent on yourself—check.

Eliminating alcohol will drastically change the way you feel on a day-to-day basis. When your sleep patterns start to normalize and your body has rebalanced after years or decades of drinking (be patient—this process can take a few weeks), you start to feel more alive every day. And who doesn't want to feel more vibrant and energetic?

When I was still drinking, I used to be envious of my dog. No, really! He was never hungover, he never felt tired after a big night, and he always woke up ready and excited to greet the day. (Side note: he was also turned off by the smell of alcohol and wouldn't go near it, like most animals. It's instinctual for them to avoid poisons. I'm sure you didn't love it the first time you tried it, but with repetition and conditioning, voilà, we become connoisseurs.) To this day, I use my dog as encouragement to wake up in the early mornings. I'll jump to him to snuggle. He's the sweetest, fluffiest Samoyed, and he's always down for cuddles, even at 5:00 a.m.

While he still beats me hands down in the energy department, my levels have dramatically changed. I feel more alive today than I ever did at twenty-one or twenty-five. My head is completely clear upon waking. No fuzziness or extra burden to carry. My body wasn't working overtime during the night to detoxify alcohol, and I feel super pampered to have slept so well instead. Behavior-change expert Andy Ramage coaches some of the top entrepreneurs and athletes in the world. He makes no qualms about it: "If you want to change your life, take a break from alcohol and improve your sleep."[1]

This good mood and outlook allow me to welcome each day as a gift. I often greet the sun and feel enthusiastic about my life. And you are meant to feel this way too. Because when it comes to getting healthy and feeling well, I know we're on the same page.

THE DETOX-JUST-TO-RETOX LOOP

I'm willing to bet you consider yourself a healthy person. Why? Because most women I work with are incredibly health-conscious. They work out on a consistent basis and aim to eat well. They value their health and are savvy to nutrition recommendations and wellness trends. Most of us do this for two reasons: we want to improve the quality of our lives, or how we feel on a day-to-day basis, and we want to live long lives. Which is why it's maddening to be stuck on the detox-just-to-retox loop that robs you of wellness. And boy, do I know this loop well, because I let this little drama play out in my life. Every. Single. Week.

You wake up, drink water with lemon, do a little stretching, and pack your green juice or salad for work. Maybe you attend a yoga class or stop by the gym on your way home. You feel so accomplished, and you've been *so* good—why not celebrate with a little wine when you get home? Except a little wine always seems to morph into two, three, or four glasses. Mark Leyshon, the senior policy and research manager at Alcohol Change UK, has said that people who exercise more also tend to drink more alcohol because they feel they've "earned it."[2] Instead of continuing on that upward spiral of well-being, you end up on the couch with Netflix, unhealthy snacks, restless sleep, and early morning disappointment, followed by straight talk that you won't drink again tonight.

My loop played out every week. On Monday mornings, disgusted and depressed with how the weekend got away from me, I resolved to be healthy and drink less. I ate the salads and had the green juice and went to workout classes. But my resolve usually crumbled around Thursday night (or Friday, if I was really holding out), and I added wine or craft beer to the equation. I always drank during the weekends, ultimately nullifying the effects of my healthy week.

If I drank too much, the next day became an excuse to eat whatever I wanted and just lounge. The irony is, today I realize you're allowed to take a day off to relax and treat yourself. But why did I have to make myself sick in order to feel I deserved it? Other times, I punished myself. Hungover or with a headache, I'd will myself to go to a workout class or, even worse, hot yoga. Ever try to sweat out the toxins? Big mistake. I almost passed out and left the yoga studio with an even bigger, more throbbing headache than when I'd arrived. Whoever passed on the idea that exercising is a great way to get rid of a hangover not only was extremely incorrect but also was recommending something very dangerous. In a hungover state, your body is so dehydrated to begin with, and working out exacerbates this.[3]

By Monday, I was emotionally depressed and felt my self-esteem crumbling. I wasn't living my life to the fullest. I made every resolution in the book and tried so hard to be good during the week. But because I felt like I'd earned it or had social events that "required" it, alcohol always showed up later in the week, followed by a weekend of drinking and back to the Monday-morning blues. Detox just to retox, over and over and over again. Maybe your loop plays out on a daily basis. Green juice in the morning and wine o'clock at night?

We accept this as a norm in our society. Alcohol companies even sponsor wellness advocates and events. Red wine is still misguidedly touted for its health benefits. Make no mistake: alcohol is no health beverage. And we're going to explore why. But you already intuitively know this, because of the way alcohol shows up in your life. You must ask yourself what the detox-just-to-retox loop does to your energy and daily mood— how you feel every day, which arguably makes up your overall quality of life. In the next chapter, I'll explain more about what alcohol does to your body on a cellular level and how it affects your major organs. Although the negative health effects of drinking are being discovered at much lower drinking levels than previously known, the science is also proving that your body can heal fast when you take a break.

UPWARD SPIRAL OF WELL-BEING

Once your body heals, I want you to imagine a different day-to-day existence: You sleep well every single night. You wake up feeling happy, proud of yourself, and enthusiastic about your day. You aren't in a bad mood, with a slight headache or brain fogginess. No racing anxiety. And that craving for fatty meals to mop up the pain goes away.

As I lived alcohol-free, I started to naturally crave healthier foods. The guilt of the night before wasn't weighing on me, and I wasn't "shoulding" all over myself about what I *should* or *shouldn't* eat. Instead, I started to eat more intuitively and naturally craved more fruits and vegetables, which boosted my mood. Studies have shown a direct correlation between happiness and fruit and vegetable intake. People who eat fruits and vegetables every day feel more optimistic and satisfied with life.[4]

You know what's even more wonderful about this effortless way of intuitive eating? I have zero guilt when I do want something more indulgent. I know my body is getting all the nutrients it needs, and I happily indulge in ice cream or cookies when I choose. I know I'm reaching for those because I genuinely want them, and eat them with a clear conscience.

Mallory, for years had saved her calories for wine and deprived herself of dessert. When she took a break from alcohol, she started to become less rigid. One Friday afternoon, she went to an ice cream shop with her family, and actually ordered something. Her daughter was ecstatic: "Mom, Mom, you got an ice cream!" It brought her family joy to experience the pleasures of life together and not replace this joy with "mommy juice" later.

You can be a lot more flexible and intuitive and still get results. Say bye-bye to yo-yo dieting once and for all. When you let go of the shoulds and transform your mindset to stop seeing alcohol as a treat (and I'll show you how), you'll stop sabotaging your health goals with wine because you "earned it."

Without the guilt or the hangovers, you'll also feel more motivated to move your body intuitively. But here's a huge tip: Don't try to change everything at once. Don't take a break and pick up veganism or commit to running five miles every day. Alcohol is what habit expert Charles Duhigg calls a *keystone habit*.[5] First, lay the foundation for an alcohol-free lifestyle, and all the other things will either fall into place or become the next focal point. Trust that removing alcohol from your routine will naturally guide you into doing the things you prioritize, including moving your body. Be gentle at first, and do what feels good to you in the moment. We'll focus on optimizing your health and healing in week three of the plan.

What would you rather have: an upward spiral of well-being and contentment or crazy, artificial spikes followed by incredible lows and anxiety? Joy and fun don't have to wait for Friday nights—they can be everyday things. Scientifically, alcohol makes you tired, cranky, low, and anxious. Not the picture of wellness, is it? Let yourself choose happy, vibrant, appreciative, well-rested, and energetic. Issa, another one of my clients, has boundless energy today. While she was always uber health-conscious before, it's stopped being something she's rigid about and started being a lot more fun. Her movement of choice? Dancing with Hula-Hoops.

CHAPTER 4

End the Weight-Loss Struggle

While going alcohol-free isn't a diet plan, you'll notice results here too. In addition to embodying more wellness in your life, many people lose weight or see their body composition change when they take a break. Personally, I struggled with losing the last ten to twenty pounds for more than a decade. My twenties were filled with so much strife over diet plans, insecurity about my body, and a lack of understanding why it was such an uphill battle to lose weight.

Before I continue this chapter, let me say that your weight and body shape don't define your worth. The number on the scale doesn't matter. I want you to love your body because you feel alive in it. I want you to feel comfortable in your skin, no matter your size. I want you to feel good and healthy. That being said, alcohol does a serious number on our metabolism and changes the way our bodies process food, and I think it's important to know this information.

. . .

A DECADE OF DIET PLANS

When I was a preteen, my mom enrolled me in ballet classes. I hated her for it at first (I was more of a tomboy growing up), but over time I fell in love with dance. By the time I was in high school, I spent most evenings in ballet class, rehearsed for shows on the weekends, danced in competitions, and went to full-time ballet school in the summers in New York City. And then I left for college. I slowed down my dancing and picked up copious amounts of drinking instead. By the time I graduated, I'd added at least twenty pounds to my frame, believing that my metabolism just sucked as I got older (never mind that I was eating pizza rolls and drinking gin and tonics like it was my job). I tried to lose some weight, but eventually I'd stop caring and go back to partying.

After UCLA, I went off to graduate school, and the problem worsened. By the time I was twenty-four, I was thirty-five pounds over my base weight. I'd scratch my head, confused that it was even possible to inflate like that, and felt at a loss when I tried to lose weight (without giving up drinking) but didn't. Thus began the never-ending diet and exercise plan I put myself on, which lasted the rest of my twenties. I fought long and hard with the weights. I did juice cleanses. I ate quinoa. I did low-carb, intermittent fasting, and high-intensity workouts. I joined a gym. I joined a yoga studio. All my effort and mental energy barely moved the needle. And when I did lose weight and keep it off, it was excruciatingly difficult.

When I got engaged at twenty-six, I finally kicked it up a notch to lose ten pounds for my wedding—so many early morning workout videos, so few carbs. Again, the number on the scale is not what defines our worth, but maybe you've struggled to lose weight too?

Since I'd become a drinker, I was on an endless quest to lose weight and eat less, and I always worried about how I looked. It was tiring. But when I stopped drinking, it finally became easy, even while eating carbs. Compared to what I'd been putting myself through for years, this felt effortless. While I had a pretty healthy lifestyle by the time I turned thirty, I didn't make any other conscious, deliberate changes, yet my body composition totally changed. I could see more muscle and less fat. And though I lost five pounds at the most, I had never felt so comfortable in my own skin. I wore whatever I wanted and felt more at home in my body. My experience trying on clothes in the dressing room completely changed. I feel better today than I have in my entire adult life. My friends tell me I look like I'm twenty.

WHY ALCOHOL CAN LEAD TO WEIGHT GAIN

I can't make any promises about how taking a break will affect your body, but I will tell you about the effect of alcohol on your metabolism and weight over time. You see, when it comes to alcohol, it's not just about calories in versus calories out. Alcohol messes with your metabolism in much more sinister ways. And other than a few wellness plans online, most gurus in the heath and diet industry barely even talk about it. Learning about these effects was a huge relief, because maybe my issues weren't solely from getting older. My complicated relationship with alcohol made weight loss so darn hard.

First of all, yes, calories do matter. Have you ever heard the diet rule "don't drink your calories"? A lot of us get the hang of this and ditch sodas, sweet fruit juices, and sugary coffee drinks. But alcohol doesn't count, right? Or we drink "light" alcohol, hoping it won't have as much of an impact. However, alcohol *does* pack on empty calories—it's the second most energy-dense (non) nutrient after fat, meaning it's high in calories and low in nutrients. One glass of wine has between 110 and 180 calories. A beer clocks in between 100 and 200. Some heavy IPAs can be 300 calories. *Three hundred calories!* That's basically a McDonald's cheeseburger. Even if you only have one a day, that's still an extra cheeseburger every day. But let's be honest. Most of us don't stop at one drink per occasion. When you routinely add 500 calories to your day, a few times a week, you can see how quickly they add up.

But other factors are working against you than just the empty calories: you also eat more when you drink alcohol because it stimulates your appetite. That explains all those greasy late-night snacks or munching on pretzels at the bar. In addition to increasing your appetite, alcohol numbs the signal telling your brain that you're full. You don't register that feeling of fullness after grazing and snacking until it's too late. Researchers from the Francis Crick Institute and University College London discovered that alcohol switches the brain into starvation mode, increasing hunger and appetite. They published their findings from a two-year investigation into how ethanol affects the body, brain, and actions of mice. Alcohol not only increased appetite but also decreased metabolism and energy levels. A similar reaction happens in humans.[1]

The ill effects don't stop there. Alcohol blocks the absorption of certain nutrients and vitamins, which then get depleted when your body is in the process of detoxifying.[2] This is mind-blowing. Most of us don't choose kale and broccoli for the taste—we eat them for those good-for-you nutrients our bodies need to be healthy. But what if your alcohol consumption sabotages these efforts? Alcohol doesn't have any vital nutrients itself, and it inhibits the absorption and usage of folic acid, zinc, and vitamins A, B, C, D, E, and K. By blocking the absorption of nutrients, alcohol yet again makes you feel hungrier because your body is missing those nutrients. Not just when you drink—alcohol makes you hungrier all the time.

Plus, now the body needs to burn off these extra calories, and it can't store alcohol as an energy source and instead has to burn it off right away. While this might sound like a good thing, it's not. We can store nutrients, protein, carbs, and fat in our body, but not alcohol. Which means your body needs to dispose of it immediately, and this takes priority over burning the calories from the food you've eaten. An *American Journal of Clinical Nutrition* study showed a 73 percent reduction in metabolism for three hours after consuming two drinks.[3] All the other macronutrients your body was supposed to burn are stored as fat instead.

Drinking alcohol seems to make losing weight an uphill battle, but what about simply working off all those extra calories and stored energy? Well, alcohol also considerably affects your ability to get physically fit. You might recall from physical education class how aerobic fitness works. You exercise your heart and muscles so that, over time, you become more efficient at pumping blood and delivering oxygen to your body. Therefore, many athletes have much lower resting heart rates. Alcohol has the exact opposite effect. It forces your heart to beat faster and increases your blood pressure, but with no related physical exertion. The heart becomes less efficient at pumping oxygen to the body, and alcohol use over time increases both heart rate and blood pressure. Not good for the cardiovascular system at all and definitely not good for getting fit—if you're looking to beat your personal best, drop alcohol and see what happens.

Alcohol also impedes muscle growth by diminishing protein synthesis, slows the body's ability to heal and recover from a workout, and depletes energy. Alcohol causes a drop in testosterone levels (needed for growing muscles) and increases cortisol.[4] So, in addition to consuming more calories, eating more, blocking nutrients, and throwing off your metabolism, add decreased energy, aerobic fitness, and muscle mass to the list.

After I learned about the ways alcohol was halting my weight-loss efforts, you know what was freeing? Realizing the problem wasn't just me. Alcohol plays a much bigger role in weight gain than common knowledge tells us. The good news is that a lot of people report weight loss results after being alcohol-free between three to six months. Please be patient, as it takes time for the body to adjust to this new normal. Some people don't lose weight but see their body composition change a bit.

Depending on your lifestyle and drinking habits, the weight loss could be quicker, slower, or not even one of your goals. Let's not forget that when you stop drinking, you also stop hangovers, lethargy, and a lack of motivation. From day to day, the benefits compound, and it's almost inevitable you'll live a healthier lifestyle.

Rebecca used to carry an extra fifty pounds on her small frame. She'd go to football games and bars with her friends and drink lots of beer and wine. She also used both alcohol and food as coping mechanisms to deal with bad days. When she looked in the mirror one day, she felt muted and like she was erasing herself. At first, her decision to take a break from alcohol was all about the weight loss. After going alcohol-free, she took up running, incorporated healthier coping mechanisms, and started working on her personal growth and voice.

She fell so in love with her new life she knew she'd never go back. You wouldn't recognize her today. She's still the life of the party, but with a mocktail in hand. She feels more like herself than ever before and is even competing in fitness competitions.

CHAPTER 5

Uplevel Your Health

HEAL YOUR BODY

While the weight loss can be wonderful, especially if it helps you feel more alive and at home in your body, much is changing on the inside too. In fact, you might be shocked at how quickly and miraculously our bodies can heal. As mentioned earlier, studies have shown that even just one month off of drinking can have massive health benefits: blood pressure and blood cholesterol decrease, liver fat improves, cancer markers go down, gray matter increases in the brain, and neurons regenerate. Plus, you're adding years to your lifespan. The positive effects of alcohol abstinence on your health add up fast. Thank heavens, because I know many of us are concerned about the damage we might have done with those bingey weekends over the years. Obviously, I'm not a doctor, nor should this information replace regular checkups and conversations with your health-care practitioner, but the science is hopeful.

As we continue to learn more about the negative effects of alcohol, as we did with smoking in recent years, I'm convinced that more experts will advise periods of abstinence, if not flat out recommending to avoid drinking altogether (the American Cancer Society already does). Unlike today, when it seems that you'd only stop drinking if you have a "problem," ditching alcohol will become a normal part of getting healthier. Wellness leaders will hop on the bandwagon, and what you're about to learn here will be common knowledge.

Right now, most doctors and wellness experts drink themselves, and the alcohol industry plays a heavy hand in studies that recommend moderation. I once read a headline about a study that recommended moderation for health reasons. Behind the glossy headline, the study design gave participants 60ml of wine one day a week. We're talking about a thimbleful of wine (three times less than what you're served in a restaurant)—in essence, proving that the least amount of wine possible is best for you. Who the heck designed this study?

While it takes time and activism to truly change a culture, we're moving in the right direction (for instance, around five million people now partake in Dry January). Until then, think of yourself as a sober rebel goddess who's doing wonders for your body. What do you have to lose? Here's what you'll reap:

Starting with the organ that drinkers worry about the most, the liver. Some people think only heavy drinking affects the liver's health, but that's not true. As craft beer and mommy juice culture dominate, doctors have seen a spike in liver issues among nonproblem drinkers over the years, especially for women and at young ages. And some of these issue have led to deaths.[1] But you can improve your liver health. A team of liver specialists found that just five weeks abstaining from alcohol decreases liver fat by 15 to 20 percent. This is great news, because fat accumulation in the liver is a prelude to liver damage.[2] The longer you're alcohol-free, the higher your chances of healing your liver back to its predrinking state.

For some reason, I wasn't concerned with liver damage, but one thing used to keep me up at night: what I was doing to my heart. I could feel it beating much faster after a drinking weekend, even to the point of feeling sore and sensing pressure on my chest. It terrified me. I couldn't understand how a twenty-something woman could have heart problems. I scoured the internet for alcohol's effects on the heart and found a lot of competing information. It turns out that alcohol misuse can lead to a heart attack—a weekend binge triples your chances of having a heart event.[3] Binge drinking also can make platelets more likely to clump together as blood clots that could lead to a heart attack.

Wait—isn't red wine good for your heart? Doesn't it lower your heart attack risk? Turns out, no, not really. The risks far outweigh any benefits, most of which were inflated due to poorly designed studies.[4] It's a thoroughly debunked misconception. The resveratrol in red wine is miniscule,[5] and a clear link indicates that drinking alcohol at any level leads to high blood pressure. One study found that less than one drink per day increased blood pressure by 1 mmHG.[6] Over time, that makes a difference. Drinking makes the heart work harder and faster, without the related physical exertion, making it less efficient at pumping blood and can eventually lead to heart failure.

Then there's the not-often-talked-about correlation between drinking and cholesterol. First off, let it sink in that more than 40 percent of American adults are worried about their cholesterol and have levels above 200,[7] and two out of every three adults either has high blood pressure or prehypertension.[8] Countless diets and exercise plans try to help people lower both of these. And if that doesn't work, doctors prescribe medication.

High blood pressure and cholesterol are crucial risk factors for heart attacks, and over time they lead to the development of atherosclerosis. If heart disease is America's number one killer, you would think we'd know that ditching alcohol or taking a break could lower both of these numbers. A study exploring the effects of Dry January showed that just five weeks of not drinking can lower blood cholesterol between ten and twenty points.[9] While alcohol doesn't have any cholesterol or saturated fat in it, it does lead to inflammation, which increases cholesterol.

I've had high cholesterol my whole adult life. I tried everything under the sun to lower it, to no avail. After nine months without drinking, I checked my cholesterol. When I got my results, I couldn't believe it: a fifty-one-point drop, from 218 (my lowest at that time) to 167. And my blood pressure decreased within a few weeks. While any amount of alcohol is found to raise blood pressure, eliminating it renders blood pressure rapidly reversible. My clients have even gotten off lifelong medications. In week 3 of the plan, I'll guide you to foods and beverages you can use to expedite these results for yourself.

Of course, drinking also impacts the brain. Drinking shrinks brain volume and can lead to cell death. Recent studies suggest that alcohol can lead to dementia and even Alzheimer's disease. In a study published in the *Journal of Neuroinflammation*, findings suggest that "alcohol inhibits the ability of microglia to efficiently clear amyloid from the brain," which contributes to a higher risk for developing Alzheimer's.[10] A recent University of Oxford study found that any amount of drinking causes damage to the brain. Let's not forget the power of habit on your brain too.[11] Reaching for a drink—after work, on Fridays, at the restaurant, whatever your cue is—leads to the development of a strong highway of neural pathways. Your brain sees the cue and automatically wants to fire neurons down that highway, thus leading to your craving.

While shrinking gray matter and neural pathways fundamentally changes the brain, studies show that within only two weeks of abstinence, gray matter starts to regrow. Between six months to a year of abstinence, it completely regenerates to predrinking levels. After a year, something really incredible happens: gray matter grows beyond where it was before ever drinking.[12] And as you change your habits and routines, neurons regenerate, new neural pathways are developed in your brain, and old ones are pruned. In other words, people who ditch drinking are more adept at self-control and have more resiliency and neuroplasticity than someone who never struggled at all.

Let's see how America's number two killer, cancer, fares with a break. In 2020, the American Cancer Society made a landmark declaration: it is best not to drink.[13] It only took thirty-two years from the time alcohol was first classified as a toxic carcinogen! Alcohol is strongly implicated in cancer—it causes more than twenty different kinds.[14] And we're not talking about heavy drinking here. Studies have proven that even two to three drinks a week increases a woman's risk of getting breast cancer by up to 15 percent.[15] *Two to three drinks a week?* That nightly glass of wine can take more of a toll than most women realize.

Want it spelled out a different way? Researchers found that for women, drinking one bottle of wine per week raises the risk of cancer as much as smoking ten cigarettes a week.[16] When I say that alcohol is the new cigarette, it's quite a literal parallel.

Don't get discouraged, though, because even with cancer, there's good news. In one study, scientists found that abstaining from alcohol for one month resulted in "a decrease in circulating concentrations of cancer-related growth factors."[17] While more long-term studies are needed to show how the risk decreases over time, you can have faith that some immediate improvements are happening.

Every year, more studies are capturing alcohol's true effects. In 2018, the largest, most comprehensive study on alcohol was published, titled, "Alcohol Use and Burden for 195 Countries and Territories, 1990–2016: A Systematic Analysis for the Global Burden of Disease Study 2016."[18] This vast report made headlines across the world, proclaiming that no level of alcohol consumption is safe. The study showed that alcohol was the cause of more than three million deaths in 2016 alone. It also showed that any amount of alcohol increased all causes of death and that one drink extra lowers your life expectancy by thirty minutes. "The health risks associated with alcohol are massive," said the senior author of the study, Dr. Emmanuela Gakidou of the Institute for Health Metrics and Evaluation at the University of Washington. "Our findings are consistent with other recent research, which found clear and convincing correlations between drinking and premature death, cancer and cardiovascular problems. Zero alcohol consumption minimizes the overall risk of health loss."[19]

When you add up all these factors, alcohol makes a huge difference to your longevity and how your body feels on a day-to-day basis. Also, let's not forget the effects alcohol has on sleep. Lack of quality sleep can lead to cancer, diabetes, depression, and daily sluggishness. From the cardiovascular improvements to the lowered risk for cancer, being alcohol-free could be the healthiest thing you can do for your body. Many of my clients see a vast improvement in their health, much better test results, and even healing from chronic issues. If the benefits of alcohol-free living were sold in a pill, pharmaceutical companies would make billions.

HEAL YOUR MIND

I can't wait for you to experience the health benefits of a break. In addition to your body healing, your mental health and daily moods will change. That alcohol affects mental health seems obvious—we understand that heavy drinkers can be depressed and even suicidal. What is much less understood is the effect of moderate but regular drinking on the brain. As you're learning, alcohol is not a benign drink. Alcohol also has strong effects on the neurochemicals in your brain, which can lead to anxiety, mild depression, and apathy.

Most people drink because they associate alcohol with a good feeling. No doubt you know what I'm talking about and have your own positive associations with drinking: feeling a nice, warm "buzz." It's true—you do receive a buzz from a drink, which usually lasts about twenty minutes and then fades. Alcohol stimulates an artificial release of dopamine in the brain, much like other drugs do. This dopamine spike peaks at a higher level than experiencing it naturally. Dopamine used to be called a happiness neurotransmitter, but now it's better classified as one that controls wanting and motivation. Our brains release dopamine when an activity is crucial to our survival, like finding and eating a piece of fruit or having sex. The dopamine is released to cement the learning—*"This behavior is important for my survival"*—and thus we learn to repeat the activity. Our brains also release glutamate to lock in this learning as a memory, so we're more apt to repeat it.[20] And because of the world we live in, we do repeat it, which continues to make the brain deem drinking as important to survival.

Not only is alcohol nonessential to our survival (just like a pack of Twizzlers isn't), the artificial dopamine spike that your brain gets from alcohol desensitizes you to dopamine and retracts your receptors.[21] So over time, certain activities that would otherwise make you feel good—for example, playing with a child or walking in the woods—aren't as enjoyable anymore because they can never compete with the dopamine that's released when you drink alcohol. You become desensitized from naturally occurring dopamine, and your brain has a new happiness threshold. Unless alcohol is involved, activities that should make or formerly made you happy don't register as high. You become neurologically unable to experience life's joys. This is why many drinkers see drinking as the epitome of experiences. Beer tasting always wins over a hike. Wine and Netflix win over stargazing.

In addition to the lowered dopamine receptivity, regular drinking lowers and depletes your levels of serotonin and GABA,[22] two neurochemicals that also make you feel happy and calm.

In the sleep chapter (chapter 2), I briefly review how the body achieves homeostasis and the way alcohol induces the release of stress hormones and stimulants. Remember: because alcohol is a depressant and slows certain functions in your body, your body tries to stabilize through the counteractive process of releasing neurochemicals like cortisol, adrenaline, dynorphin, and corticotropin-releasing factor. Studies show that the longer you're a drinker, the more these stress hormones circulate in your body after drinking. This is true even after just a few glasses.[23] It also takes days for these hormones to stop circulating in your body. They can make you feel overanxious, apathetic, or sad, or have racing thoughts. The anxiety and tension can feel like you're on edge all the time.

Subconsciously, a lot of drinkers look forward to drinking, because it gives them momentary relief from being on edge. So, we drink to remove the side effects that drinking brought on in the first place! (When there's no edge, drinking doesn't feel as good: drinkers who start drinking again after a long break often don't get the same relief as when they're in the cycle.) In addition to tricking your mid- and lower-brain into thinking alcohol is important to your survival, these stimulants help explain why it's easy to grab another drink after the first one. When the initial twenty-minute buzz wears off and your blood-alcohol level falls, you feel the uncomfortable side effects. Hence, you reach for a drink to trigger another spike and avoid the crash. Plus, because alcohol slows your prefrontal cortex, it prohibits sound judgment and decision-making. Don't simply chalk up your inability to stop at one drink as a lack of self-control. This is how alcohol is meant to interact with your brain.

Drinking used to leave me with a cloud of negativity, anxiety, and exhaustion. After a weekend of drinking, it took a few days to feel normal again. It wasn't me though—it was a chemical cocktail in my brain that twisted my feelings, emotions, and moods. I didn't think of myself as a depressed or anxious person, so I kept all my post-drinking lows to myself. We often discount this experience and only associate the first twenty minutes, the buzz, with alcohol. Yet drinking is a forty-eight-hour experience, during which your body and brain work overtime to repair and recalibrate. Take notice next time. Are you more prone to anxiety, racing thoughts, frustration, disappointment, crankiness, and exhaustion after drinking? If so, don't disregard this.

While many people drink after work to help relieve stress, alcohol scientifically does the opposite to both your body and brain—alcohol creates stress. There is a connection between alcohol and anxiety on a molecular level, as one study demonstrated.[24] While life on the other side isn't necessarily all sunshine and rainbows, week five of the plan will dive deep into improving your mental health and discuss healthier alternatives for dealing with stress and anxiety.

The effects of alcohol on your brain chemistry can last weeks, meaning that most regular drinkers have no idea what their natural state feels like. It takes about four to six weeks for your brain chemistry to rebalance and, at this benchmark, many people feel a surge of positive feelings and joy, with glimmers of a natural buzz gifted in life's most beautiful moments. I hadn't gone a few weeks without alcohol since I was a teenager. When I took a break, I remember being amazed by clouds and trees, belting out songs in my car, and having dance parties with my dog. I hadn't felt that euphoric since the last time I'd fallen in love.

HOW YOU LOOK

And all of this positivity shows in your appearance as well. Ready to look more radiant than you have in years? Within weeks, if not days, the brightness of your skin and eyes will greatly improve. "Alcohol is actually one of the worst, most aggressive compounds to destroy your skin," says New York nutritionist Jairo Rodriguez. "I always joke with my patients, 'If you want to get older, go ahead and drink!'"[25] Point blank: Drinking ages you. Along with causing your body to hold on to extra weight, alcohol makes your face puffy and bloated. It dries out your skin, and it can lead to redness and broken capillaries. Alcohol breaks down collagen, gives you more wrinkles, and makes you look older than you are. It reddens and yellows your eyes or dulls them to look lifeless. And since alcohol disrupts sleep, drinking can also lead to dark circles, paleness, and a look of exhaustion. Compare the appearance of drinkers to nondrinkers, and you'll see a difference.

Before-and-after photos always astound me. Sometimes I can't believe I'm looking at the same person. And you're in for a surprise too. In the eight-week plan, we'll take comparison selfies, so you can see the difference for yourself. I bet your skin will look better, your eyes will be bright, and you will look more at peace. I took a photo of myself at the end of sixty days alcohol-free, and I was shocked. My face! I saw an eagerness and brightness to my face I hadn't seen since I was a little girl. I could see the six-year-old version of myself in my face, and her innocent optimism brought me to tears. I was glowing from within.

My client Lisa came to me with blotchy red skin, puffiness under her eyes, and a look of perpetual exhaustion. Two months into her journey, her skin was glowing and her eyes sparkled, and she looked at least five years younger. If you spend money on creams and treatments to prevent aging, why not just try a break from alcohol instead? If you care about looking radiant, young, and vibrant, this book can help you look better than you have in years. The skin can rehydrate and regenerate with a break from alcohol, which may become your new favorite beauty secret.

Quick health benefits of an eight-week break:

- Brain gray-matter grows and neurons regenerate
- Neurochemicals rebalance
- Sleep improves
- Liver heals
- Blood pressure and cholesterol go down
- Cancer markers decrease

- Weight loss occurs
- Appearance improves

THE MONEY YOU SAVE

Let's not sugarcoat it: drinking is expensive. While you might think you spend a little here and a little there, because alcohol is often a nonnegotiable (almost like food), the money adds up. HuffPost calculated that the average drinker spends between $2,500 and $7,800 a year on alcohol.[26] I've probably wasted tens of thousands of dollars over my lifetime. On alcohol alone. I can't even imagine how many ancillary costs would add on top of that: cab and Uber rides, fourth meals, and items lost.

You could save a small fortune by redirecting your alcohol costs to something you really want in your life. If you're used to going out to bars, breweries, pubs, or gastropubs, that's an immediate, huge savings. Consider your grocery bill—no bottles of wine, no twelve-packs, no liquor. Your grocery bill is bound to be much less. The money savings show up in less obvious places too. Have you ever been to a high-end restaurant and not ordered a drink to go with your meal? You know, a painstakingly expensive seventeen-dollar cocktail or severely overpriced glass of wine? Those hurt. I remember so many nice dinners out when I was younger. I'd nurse one pricey drink, angry that I wasn't rich enough to buy another. Instead of being in the moment and enjoying my date, I couldn't wait to go home and have another, cheaper drink.

Drinking at any special occasion inevitably increased the bill by at least forty dollars. And that was when my husband and I were being frugal. Imagine the cost of a bottle of wine or a few drinks. We always tried to order the least expensive food item but never thought to part with our cocktails. Ditto anyplace you're accustomed to buying drinks: concerts, horse races, amusement parks, networking events, cruises, vacations. With one decision, you cut out all that extra pain and discomfort—discomfort that comes from needing a drink in any given situation (like a dinner outing) and the pain that comes with having to swallow a hefty bill. It's incredibly freeing!

All that money can go into savings or be spent guilt-free on things that make you happy. For instance, how about ordering dessert at the fancy restaurant? Not only have I saved thousands of dollars since going alcohol-free, but I have also radically changed my money mindset. For years, I wanted this thirty-dollar face cream, but it seemed like too much money and too frivolous of a purchase. But a thirty-dollar brewery tab? That was a normal expense. I made these kinds of justifications for alcohol all the time. Think about it: Have you ever spent more than sixty bucks on alcohol in one night? If you could buy something you've always wanted within that price range, what would you get? I could get a new jacket, a massage, three new books, a chef's tasting menu, a learning seminar, or a new perfume. And these are all things that will bring me more joy and pampering than a half-remembered night at a bar. The savings compound, and you start to define a new normal of treating yourself—in a way that's aligned with your actual desires.

PART II
Your Mind and Soul

CHAPTER 6

Uncover Your Limiting Beliefs

YOUR BELIEFS EITHER EMPOWER OR DISEMPOWER YOU

Would you believe me if I told you that most of your behavior results from the beliefs you have? I'm not talking about religious beliefs, but rather the things you either consciously or subconsciously believe to be true. Studies have shown that our beliefs can affect how fast we heal, how we respond to medical treatment (ever heard of the placebo effect?), how we perform on standardized tests, and how successful we become. Our beliefs aren't facts—they're assumptions. They're drawn from external events and people and then filtered and distorted in our brain, according to our past experiences, upbringing, values, and emotional state. Your beliefs color your reality and shape your thoughts, feelings, behavior, and results. You view the world through your beliefs, and you act them out. In essence, they determine your destiny.

Every belief you have either empowers you or limits you. If you've ever read a personal development book, you may be familiar with the term *self-limiting beliefs*. Whether you're conscious of it or not, you have beliefs that do not serve you and your growth. And that's the thing: most of our beliefs are subconscious and run our lives on autopilot—especially beliefs surrounding alcohol.

According to the National Science Foundation, we have more than 60,000 unique thoughts a day. Eighty percent of our daily thoughts are negative, and 95 percent are repeat thoughts.[1] The key to transforming your relationship with alcohol is transforming thoughts and beliefs you might not even know you have.

In the eight-week plan I share later in the book, I'll walk you through the exact process to address your self-limiting beliefs. You'll learn how to notice the belief, question whether it serves you and your success, and if it doesn't, how to erase and replace it. Much of the time, we believe things about alcohol that aren't scientifically true.[2] Other times, we think we need a drink to access a state we don't believe we're capable of achieving on our own. You are far more powerful than you may realize. And you get to choose what to believe! You might as well give yourself every chance to pursue what you truly want in this lifetime.

CHANGE YOUR MINDSET: FEEL LUCKY INSTEAD OF DEPRIVED

Many people try to take a break or quit drinking by solely changing their behavior. Maybe you've tried this too. You say you won't drink for a week or a few days. You muster all your willpower to constantly say no to yourself. This approach doesn't feel very good, does it? Definitely not "euphoric." While positive behavior change is great, it can leave a vacuum of deprivation behind, and you may feel like you're always missing out.

I've met people who've been sober for a while, even for years, yet still pine for alcohol. I don't want you to live this way. And the solution is much simpler than you might think. When you change your mindset (that is, beliefs), you can arrive at a place where you don't want to drink anymore. Where the activity loses its allure. Where you feel lucky to be a nondrinker. As the Buddhist teaching goes, when there is no desire, there is no suffering.

Consciously, you probably want to drink less or not at all. That's why you're reading this book. But subconsciously, you crave alcohol. You still want to pour a drink on a Friday at 5:00 p.m. or have a glass of wine when you're out with your friends. It's almost as if two parts of your brain are at war with each other—a result of cognitive dissonance. It's extremely painful to live in this state. As long as you believe that drinking holds some benefits, comfort, or mystique, you'll continue to crave it, despite its negative effects. You'll continue to feel like you're missing out if you don't drink.

I lost my desire for alcohol within a few months of my alcohol-free journey. And I didn't land there by accident. I was ruthless. I had to uncover every single reason I liked to drink in the first place, hold up each and every belief for scrutiny, and then find new beliefs to replace the old ones. I have hundreds of pages of journaling I did during this time, while I was questioning, learning, and peeling back the layers of the onion. I'm so glad I did, because it allowed me to lose my desire for alcohol for good and feel ecstatic about it. Which is pretty crazy for me, considering that I'd been drinking regularly since I was seventeen and thought it was my favorite pastime.

In weeks 1 and 4 of the eight-week plan, we'll go step by step to uncover your limiting beliefs around alcohol and the process you need to overturn them or let them go. In my coaching practice, I've walked hundreds of women through this process, and most of the beliefs are surprisingly common. And how do I identify these subconscious beliefs? I simply ask my clients why they like to drink.

Suffice it to say, this mindset work is worth it. And you don't have to toil over it with hundreds of pages of journaling. I did the hard work for you and will be sharing my exact framework with you, to get the mental freedom you deserve—because you were made to use your beautiful mental energy and intellect on much more meaningful gifts to this world.

IS THE BELIEF SCIENTIFICALLY TRUE?

One of my biggest reasons for drinking and the most common thing I hear from clients is this: it helps me relax. Said another way: it helps me unwind. Said another way: it helps me shut down my overactive brain. Said another way: it helps me turn off my racing thoughts. Whenever I work with a client and start to uncover these kinds of beliefs, I filter them through two different questions: Is this belief scientifically true? Does this belief empower or disempower you?

First, is this belief scientifically true? As your brain gets intoxicated, alcohol is slowing down the prefrontal cortex, the speed at which your neurons fire, and the ability to think critically. Alcohol has been used as an anesthetic for centuries. If it does one thing effectively, it numbs. It numbs or suppresses your thoughts, feelings, and emotions in a short time frame. We've all seen the negative side of this effect when buzzed becomes drunk, and you can't think clearly.

But like I always say to my clients, drinking isn't a twenty-minute buzz or even a few hours of numbness. It's a forty-eight-hour experience. As you learned earlier, in the chapters on sleep (chapter 2) and how alcohol affects your neuro-chemicals (chapter 5), alcohol induces the release of stress hormones in your body and unleashes waves of anxiety and racing thoughts. It's common to feel this effect most acutely the next day.

In reality, drinking is like putting your head in the sand for a few hours while the waves crash down around you. Alcohol creates anxiety, racing thoughts, rumination, recrimination, and decision fatigue. And it doesn't even have to wait for the next day to hit you. Once I started drinking, my monkey mind, or racing thoughts, went into overdrive. *Do I have wine teeth? Should I have another? Oh, but I was supposed to wake up early to-morrow. Maybe one more wouldn't hurt. But I really shouldn't.* The next day: *Oh, god, not again. Just have one, you said! Why is this so hard? Ugh, I just want to sleep in and disappear. But I have the pre-sentation today. I can't believe I did this again.* A day later: *Should I drink tonight? I told myself I wouldn't, but won't it look weird if I don't? And it is Friday. Okay, but just one. Yeah, but you never stick to just one. Tonight I will!*

Drinking doesn't have to look like an episode out of the reality TV show *Intervention* to drain your mental energy. Being sick of the mental gymnastics—the internal games, scheming, and arguments—is one of the most common reasons women seek to change their relationship with alcohol. Mental gymnas-tics and relaxation don't go hand in hand.

When you're aware of your reasons for drinking, you can hold them up to the light and see if they pass the test of truth. Many innocuous reasons you might like to drink attach a qual-ity to alcohol that isn't scientifically true. A blaring example is the belief that alcohol helps you sleep. Alcohol is one of the worst sleep disrupters. You might believe that alcohol relaxes you and slows down your racing thoughts. Alcohol is giving you racing thoughts in the first place! Become analytical about this. Alcohol doesn't truly relax you. If anything, it gives you permission to turn off your brain for a while, but the next day, you often feel even more stressed and anxious than if you hadn't imbibed. Alcohol not only induces your body to release stress hormones, it also inhibits your ability to manage stress. For example, when I drank to relieve stress or relax, instead I could have written to-do lists, processed my feelings by journaling, or done things to relax that make me feel more grounded and accomplished, like working out, doing yoga, or a relaxing nightly routine. But back then, I decided to drink and would wake up feeling worse.

DOES THE BELIEF SERVE YOU?

Next, you can examine whether the thought or belief serves you. Does it empower you or disempower you? Does it make you feel capable, powerful, and limitless, or does the belief lean on alcohol like a crutch? We give alcohol way too much credit. We think it helps us achieve a state we're incapable of reaching on our own. You are more than just capable of achieving these states on your own. *You are powerful beyond measure.*

As a lifelong introvert, I outsourced all my confidence and fun to alcohol. I believed it turned me into a social butterfly and made me more charming. (Have we had a drunk conversation before? If so, I'm sorry.) These beliefs kept me stuck in a pattern that didn't serve me and limited my own power. If I believed that drinking made everything more fun, did that mean that deep down I thought life was boring and incredibly dull? If I believed that drinking made me more charming and likable, did that mean I believed I was uninteresting and unworthy of being liked without a chemical flowing through my veins? Both of these thoughts are kind of sad. And I was largely unaware that these beliefs were underneath my relationship with alcohol until I started to uncover them.

Once you uncover your beliefs, you need to prove them false. You can't do that unless you test them. Back when I thought drinking made me more confident and made socializing easier, I upheld that belief in a confirmation bias loop. I rarely tested the alternative or was quick to dismiss it. On the outset, it might appear that alcohol gives you liquid courage and allows you to be more outgoing. However, continually outsourcing your sociability to alcohol means you never develop that skill within yourself. It's like a muscle that never gets worked out. Of course I didn't feel confident socializing without a drink—I'd never practiced!

I used to be really insecure, and to tell you the truth, I wasn't that confident even with a drink. I constantly worried about how I appeared and sounded. *Was I too buzzed? Did I have wine teeth? Did they notice I poured a third?* If I got drunk, regardless of what happened, I felt *so* embarrassed the next day. I ruined many evenings because of this misguided belief that alcohol made me more confident. It left me with more embarrassments, more insecurities, and less of a healthy sense of self. Saying I needed a drink to socialize completely discounted me—it stripped me of my natural abilities to connect with other human beings. I gave myself too little credit. Sure, at first I was nervous socializing without a drink, but that's part of being a human! Many of us feel awkward in social situations. Learn to overcome this challenge, and you'll feel proud that you did.

As you work through all the reasons you like to drink, debunk them one at a time with alternate evidence. You'll chip away at your desire for alcohol until you're left with no desire at all. Because if you believe alcohol has no benefits, even subconsciously, you won't want to drink anymore. It will lose its allure, putting you in the driver's seat of your life and in total control of your choices.

CHAPTER 7

When You Let Yourself Down

You probably don't need me to tell you how emotionally taxing the mental gymnastics are, because it's not just frustrating and confusing, it's also incredibly painful. When you fall short of your expectations or the image of who you want to be in this world, it hurts. It erodes your self-esteem and makes you feel like you aren't enough as you are. And then there's the shame, one of the most isolating and lonely feelings in the world. When I constantly used to let myself down, it made me think I was the only person struggling and that I was somehow broken.

FEELING ASHAMED

Shame is a ubiquitous human emotion. It makes us feel small, stupid, and worthless. When we experience shame, we tend to hide our experience and bury our emotions. Even a relatively benign and harmless shame-inducing experience—like flubbing a word while public speaking or during an interview—allows feelings of inadequacy to fester and grow.

Shame holds you back from being expressive, unapologetic, and expansive. I lived in my private shame cave for years. And I wish that someone had been there to coax me out.

When alcohol distorts your ability to think clearly, embarrassing missteps are bound to happen. Has anyone ever told you what happened the night before and you just can't even? While I might have laughed it off in front of my husband or whatever friend or family member was there, for the next few days, I smoldered in shame. I didn't want to show my face anywhere and tried to avoid anything to do with the night in question. When I got way too drunk, I stopped asking what I'd done the night before because I didn't want to know. And telling myself "never again" was a lie. I couldn't say with certainty that these situations wouldn't repeat themselves. Drinking too much led to humiliating, inauthentic behavior that created more soul-crushing shame.

Take one of my best friends' bachelorette parties. It was one year before I ditched alcohol for good, so I was already trying hard to be mindful about drinking. I didn't want to go on a daylong binge and later feel ashamed and stupid. My friend planned the party at an outdoor spa, followed by dinner and a sleepover. I told myself I wouldn't drink until later in the day, and I hoped to relax at the spa, maybe take a yoga class, and stay connected with my friends. Instead, I arrived to our hotel at 11:00 a.m. to goblets of champagne and tequila shots.

Not wanting to feel left out or like a stick in the mud, I obliged. By noon, I'd had two wine goblets full of champagne, two shots of tequila, and even brought more tequila with me to the spa, so I wouldn't have to buy drinks there (I used to think this kind of strategy was smart). I ended up blacking out before I even got out of the Uber when we arrived at the spa— where I spent the next four hours doing god knows what and sleeping on a lawn chair. To this day, I have no idea what the spa looked like, but Google tells me there were waterfalls and mud baths.

I still shudder at the memory of that weekend. It's a perfect example of how my carefully laid plans often unraveled and imploded. (On the flip side, I was more mindful and drank way less at my own bachelorette party.) Alcohol is sneaky and behaves like a toxic boyfriend. One minute he loves you, and the next moment he utterly disrespects you—leaving you confused and trying hard to figure out the right thing to do or say.

Shame exists on much smaller playing fields too. Maybe you already have boundaries you won't cross. Only drink two or three drinks, but on more evenings than you wish. You might try to limit it to one drink or to have more nondrinking nights per week. Yet anytime you set an intention—for example, only have one drink tonight—and you break that intention, even by one drink, you create feelings of shame and add to your evidence list of reasons why you think you can't trust yourself.

Instead of ever believing I was awesome and should go for awesome things in my life, I was hiding and telling myself how unqualified, unreliable, insignificant, and dumb I was. Maybe not consciously, but subconsciously, the shame I never learned to let go of held me back. Even if I could forget about something idiotic I'd done in 2010, I had no guarantee that on any given weekend, I wouldn't have three beers and stupidly start a fight with my husband and feel that hot shame again.

Because of all the expectations placed on women to be perfect and excel at home, in their career, and in motherhood, moms can carry an extra load of internal shame. My client Rachel was doing all the right things. She was active in her community, had a great career, and took care of her family of three. And yet, when she drank around her kids, she was taken further away from the mom she wanted to be. She felt herself lose any sense of mindful presence, and her patience vanished. The night became about hurrying them to bed and feeling snappish. That's not how she wanted to make memories. She felt she was not only letting herself down continually, but also her kids. She didn't want them to see wine as her way to get through raising them. Forgiving herself in week 2 of Become Euphoric™ released a lot of pain for her, and today she's proud of who she is, inside and out.

LETTING GO OF SHAME

So, how do you let go of shame? Research professor and legend Brené Brown says it best: "Shame hates it when we reach out and tell our story."[1] The antidote to shame is vulnerability. Part of the reason my shame was so smoldering hot and painful was because I never ever talked about it with another soul. I could talk about, share, and then get over other missteps in my life, but I kept anything to do with drinking locked away. Such secrecy impedes our ability to be honest with ourselves and feel truly aligned with our authenticity. It also validates the idea that parts of us are unacceptable and need to be disowned and unacknowledged. However, you are the entirety of the human experience. You've done bad things and have had bad things happen to you. You also have a tender heart and truly care. You are a perfectly imperfect human who is here to learn, grow, and evolve.

My recipe for letting go of shame, which you'll learn about in week 2 of the plan, looks like this: Own your truth + Accept yourself + Forgive. By doing this in a community with others, you'll know that you've never been alone. Every day I get messages from people who share with me a discontent that they've been keeping secret for too long, and I applaud them for it. It's a relief to share and let it go off your heart, and I'm honored to hold that space for them.

If you'd like a head start on giving voice to the parts of yourself you're not entirely proud of in order to heal, I'd love to invite you to join the private Euphoric community, filled with soul-seekers who are rooting for you. You can access the link to join in the bonuses for this book at www.euphoricaf.com/book-bonus.

STAYING STUCK HURTS

We're here on planet Earth to grow—emotionally, spiritually, intellectually, and in courage. Everything in our known universe is doing one of two things: either slowly growing or slowly dying. There is no in-between or standing still in nature. It's normal for kids and young adults to explore the world, learn lessons, and mature. When you stop growing as an adult because you're stuck in a rut or using alcohol to manage your emotions, it means you're never feeling and thus not learning from them. It also means you're never challenging yourself outside your comfort zone and therefore not growing. Sleepwalking through life is no way to live. You're not here to just get by, just work the nine-to-five, just pay the bills, just raise the kids. You have passions and a purpose inside of you that are meant to be expressed. Staying stuck not only limits who you truly are; it also perpetuates an unhealthy coping mechanism to bury the fact that you're stuck in the first place. Drinking and unfulfillment go hand in hand. You owe it to yourself to find a true sense of fulfillment.

CHAPTER 8

Grow Your Self-Esteem and Confidence

The process of dismantling limiting beliefs around alcohol and healing the shame and pain around letting yourself down does something incredible for your mind. It declutters it by absolving a host of negative beliefs and feelings and freeing up space—space for you to redevelop positive beliefs about yourself and welcome more love, self-esteem, and confidence into your life. And as you take a break from alcohol, you'll find those feelings blossoming, along with your sense of integrity and pride.

While *self-love* is a word that may be thrown around a lot these days, it really does extend to more than liking your body parts. Self-love is grounded in taking care of yourself, in aligning your life to your deeper values, so you feel a sense of integrity. Drinking culture, much like diet culture, is meant to erode your self-esteem. There's no denying it: Alcohol creates pain. Whether it's the cumulative effects of letting yourself down, or all the shitty things that can happen when your inhibitions are down and your prefrontal cortex is impaired, being a drinker inevitably comes with baggage. Let's take a look at how a break helps you grow a healthy sense of self.

SELF-ESTEEM

When you say one thing or make an intention and then completely break it, you not only feel let down, you feel like you can't trust yourself. And then you vow it will be different next time, but it's not. It keeps happening and slowly erodes your self-esteem. You don't trust that you can keep promises to yourself. They almost become meaningless. Maybe you don't let yourself think about it too often, but you can't escape the wash of honesty that hits you at 4:00 a.m., waking you up with a racing heart and a knot in the pit of your stomach. Maybe that honesty is a simple fact: *I don't sleep well after any amount of wine.* Most women I work with obviously feel unwell after they have three or four glasses but also feel lousy after one or two. It's a no-win situation.

And without even consciously realizing it, this erosion of your self-esteem also erodes your sense of possibility and change. Your inner critic gets louder, and you feel more defeated. If you can't even manage this part of your life, what makes you think you can do anything else? But you can repair your self-esteem. It can happen magically when you take a break from alcohol because you fundamentally take care of yourself—you give yourself the gift of self-love.

SELF-LOVE

Have you ever taken care of yourself or a situation so that in the future, you'd have a better experience? Imagine things like washing your sheets or cleaning the house before a vacation. It feels so good to come home to clean sheets or a clean house! Sometimes it's doing things today so you don't have problems later, like flossing to prevent dental issues or taking care of an annoying administrative errand. You might not feel like flossing tonight, but the future version of you will be much happier not to suffer a root canal. You might not want to wash the sheets, but future you will love sleeping in warm, lavender-scented linen.

Drinking me didn't care about future me. She had no regard for future me. All she cared about was what felt fun and good in the moment—*One more couldn't hurt!* Or worse, *Whatever, I'll just be hungover tomorrow—I'll deal with it then.* Then future me woke up after the rough sleep with a headache and no motivation to tackle the day. *Didn't the past version of me know any better? Why didn't she care about how I'd feel?* Every time I woke up after that version of me was in control, it was painful and depressing. *How could she have been so stupid? Why didn't she think to stop at two drinks? Didn't she know how I would feel? Didn't she care?* I felt so unloved. So uncared for. And so disrespected. It's pretty obvious that I didn't feel deep and lasting love for myself. Hell, I couldn't even trust myself.

Now that I don't have that destructive habit anymore, I have regained so much love and respect for myself. Self-love means I am looking out for future me. Going to bed without drinking might feel weird on your first few nights, but there's no doubt about it: Morning you will love you for it. Because when you wake up the next day, you will feel cared for, respected, and loved by the past version of you. One of my favorite things is to wake up feeling good in the morning, and I'm thankful to this day that the past version of me has the foresight to ensure I wake up feeling loved. I feel grateful to yesterday me. My intentions were honored. I am looking out for future me when

I exercise and eat nutritious food. I know that it makes me feel my best and uplifts my mood, plus offers long-term benefits for my health. I am looking out for future me when I take care of situations that need handling. I know that the future me will be grateful the errands were run, the finances handled. Because when I fast-forward in time, I feel cared for by the past version of me, like we are on the same team.

Not drinking alcohol is the most radical act of self-love I can think of. It allows you to become aware of your inner life and take care of your needs in healthy ways. What you do every day builds who you become. This type of self-love evolves you. When you truly take care of yourself, you love yourself. Self-care isn't just about taking bubble baths (although I do love baths!). And wine is definitely not self-care. Regularly showing yourself love like this also creates a healthy sense of integrity.

INTEGRITY

Missing the mark on who I wanted to be ruined my sense of integrity. Sure, there were big ways I missed the mark. But it was the littlest things that got to me. I used to have a 50 percent chance of brushing my teeth on any given night that I drank. Yep, I was a thirty-year-old, grown-ass adult who didn't brush her teeth at night. Forget flossing. That rarely ever happened (drinking or not). When I was in a *hangxiety*, that super-emotional and anxious state after drinking, I could hardly keep up with the bare minimum of life. I couldn't be bothered. If my parents called me, there was no way I was calling them back. I lost my integrity when I snoozed on my self-development and instead just hoped my life would improve. I felt like a dimmed version of me, not expressing what it meant to be intrinsically me, not working toward my higher good. Drinking and post-drinking me was a shell of the person I wanted to be.

What does all of this have to do with integrity? Integrity is acting congruently and consistently with your deeper values and moral code. Integrity in your personal growth means you strive to show up as the person you want to be in this world. It's not about being perfect. It's about trying, not shrugging off or hiding. In what ways did I fail to show up and be the kind of person I always wanted to be? I always wanted to be the kind of person who brushes her teeth at night, for one. I always wanted to be a daughter who honored, respected, and loved her parents and was there for them in their elder years. You know, the kind of person who calls her parents back.

I always wanted to be the kind of wife who bonds with her husband and cherishes their time together, instead of the kind who has to ask upon waking, "What happened last night?" The kind who doesn't embarrass him by drinking too much. The kind who doesn't have droopy eyelids and no idea how unconnected she is. I always wanted to be the kind of aunt who's present with her niece and setting an example of self-love, instead of one who shows inauthentic affection to her (while buzzed) or disengages. I hated drinking around children and teenagers. What was I modeling to them? It bothered me a lot. With adults, everyone's bought into this social code. But with kids, I had to ask myself, *What do they think when they see me reach for another glass? What do they think when I become a dimmed version of me?*

How about that past version of me, who almost never wrote? Who dreamed of being a writer but didn't participate in the practice of writing? All I ever wanted was to be a writer, yet drinking me couldn't muster the time or energy to do it. The chasm between who I wanted to be and how I showed up in the world was huge.

Giving alcohol the boot was the key to getting my integrity back. It's given me the mood and energy to do the right things. No shame, no regrets, no Jekyll-and-Hyde behavior holds me back. Because I'm alcohol-free, drinking more than I want to is no longer as issue. I call my parents back. I brush my teeth, floss, and remove my makeup every single night. I bond with my husband and devote attention to our quality time. I play and laugh with my niece and nephew, with no fears that I'm modeling unhealthy coping skills or destructive habits. I write. I journal. I use my pen and paper almost daily. I finally wrote a book, and I call myself a writer. I'm using my unique talents and gifts every single day as a coach and teacher. Every day, I show up and try to be the kind of person I want to be.

I'm not perfect; I'll never be perfect. Sometimes I don't feel like showing up, and that's okay, too, but I spend the majority of my time in the game. When I was drinking, I spent so much time isolated and in hiding, ultimately withdrawing from my life. Instead, I jealously watched how others built their dream lives, while I complained about mine. Integrity looks like living your life in alignment with your values, not just wishing you did. I don't just say the words. I show myself how much I care, how much I love myself. I show it with my actions.

PRIDE

Pride can be a two-sided coin. There's the stubborn kind of pride—the "I can do it all on my own," bootstraps kind of pride. I've always been a prideful person who never wanted to let on that alcohol (or anything) affected me in a negative way. I tried so hard, so valiantly, and so privately, to figure out the elusive balance and make it work for me. From the mental gymnastics and rules to constantly berating myself, it took up a lot of mental space.

For a moment, I want to point out how absurd this is. I was living in a constant state of disappointment over a beverage. A beverage! An inanimate thing! Can you imagine if advanced aliens were watching our planet and noticed how many people struggled and lived in mediocrity because of a beverage? These wise and intelligent beings would have swift advice: Clearly the beverage is bringing you down—remove it from your life immediately and avoid it, like you would rattlesnakes or toxic boyfriends or anything else that is primed to harm you. They would have no qualms about this, no logical reasoning and scheming about why this beverage needs to be protected. No mental gymnastics to show how you can not only survive but endure rattlesnake bites, but you know, moderately.

I clung to pride to prove to the world that I was okay and could handle my business. And many of the women I work with feel the exact same way. It's as if deciding to change your relationship with alcohol means you are admitting defeat and weakness. And that trying to make it work in your life is some misguided way to defeat it. Somehow, these are the only two options presented to us, so rather than admit defeat, we gear up, we train, we go through the mental gymnastics. We spend all this time, our mental energy, trying to beat it. It's like being stuck in a boxing ring: You against alcohol. Sometimes you win. Sometimes he wins. You keep training and going back to fight. And while win or get defeated may seem like the only two options when you're panting in the ring, I want you to zoom out. Zoom out of the boxing ring. Zoom out of the grimy basement gym where you've been training. Look outside. Go walk in the park and breathe in some beautiful fresh air. To defeat your foe, you don't have to spend your life training and fighting in that grimy gym. You can stay outside and travel the world! Walking away from alcohol isn't losing against him. It's acknowledging that you have far better things to do with your time and your life. That you are made for more, and your beautiful mental energy is better used to create a life you love.

I carried way too much stubborn pride and thought for far too long that making changes was admitting defeat. So, instead of going after what I really wanted in my life, I settled for the status quo and hated myself for it. But when I got out of my microcosm, I realized life isn't merely A or B—it also could be C, D, E, F, and on to Z. I could transform my relationship with alcohol and didn't have to attach a label or a story of what that act means about me. Except for the story about self-love. That doing right by me, for me, for my well-being, for my growth, for my potential and purpose, were the only reasons that mattered.

The pride that held me back started to become the pride that propelled me forward. When you take a break from alcohol, the days accomplished feel like such a feat. Because each milestone is stretching you further than you've ever been. It's like running. The first time you run two miles, you beam with pride. Move it up to five miles, and you think you're superwoman. Run a half-marathon race, and you've just joined the ranks of the gods. The first two weekends you don't drink: *Oh, hello, look at me.* You get to twenty-one days: *Yes, yes, yes!* Thirty days: *Can you believe it?* Fifty days: *Who in the world is this person? Who doesn't drink for fifty days?* A hundred days: *I'm superwoman and can do anything.*

And then there are the events. The first time you don't drink at a party or a cookout, you wake up feeling amazing and feel sorry for everyone who drank. Your first wedding, your birthday, your first vacation, every single new occasion and milestone are chances to celebrate the hell out of yourself. You do the thing you said you'd do, this hard and unique thing most people won't do, the thing you've never done before, and you're smashing it! You feel faith in yourself again. You believe. You feel like a goddess rock star. You're a huge accomplishment, and you're beaming because of it.

CONFIDENCE

And all that pride in doing something you've never done before starts working on your confidence. Add to it your new radiant appearance, energy, Zen-like calm, and euphoric happiness, and you're a brand-new person walking down the street. You are beautiful, intelligent, intuitive, and an inspiration. If you can do this, what else can you do?

The thing most of us get wrong about confidence is believing it's a naturally occurring feeling or some kind of innate personality characteristic. It's neither. Confidence is the result of taking action and gaining competence. If you wait for confidence before you dare to try something new, you'll be waiting forever. The secret is in the action. In feeling the fear and doing it anyway. And the very act of taking a break from alcohol is a massive leap of action that builds your confidence in many ways. You start challenging yourself and pushing yourself beyond your limits. Ten days, twenty-one days, fifty days. Who is this new you? And what else could she do if she put her mind to it?

CHAPTER 9

Become Present to Your Beautiful Life

These days, mindfulness gets a lot of hype, for good reason. Perhaps you've meditated or gone to yoga classes or simply know that life happens way too fast and there's value in slowing down and enjoying all the beautiful moments that make it up.

For years I made new years' resolutions to meditate more often, so I could train my brain to be blissfully aware to the here and now. Except my drinking habits made it almost impossible to be mindful, and instead created a state of mindlessness. I lived for the weekend. Happiness was always just a drink away. I was always anticipating a better reward. When I was wishing time could go faster, to the next weekend, to the next drink, to the time that my hangover would subside, I never realized I was basically wishing *my life* would go faster. When I felt lousy, the day was a chore, and I couldn't wait for it to be over. I wanted to press fast-forward. I was wishing my life away instead of being intentional about creating a life from which I didn't want to escape. Wednesday night was nice, but Friday night would be even better, when I could enjoy some wine.

The way alcohol manipulates dopamine means it creates anticipation in the brain, drastic artificial peaks to look forward to. And nothing quite compares with those peaks. Of course, this isn't a direct experience—it's deeply subconscious, meaning you don't quite realize why you don't feel comfortable inside your skin.

WONDER AND AWE

Many years ago, I was on a waterfall hike with my husband. The path followed a stream in a canyon that created this magical forest grove to walk through. I live in San Diego, known for its chaparral, and this hike was otherworldly with its lush forest and water. Intellectually, I knew how beautiful all of this was, but I couldn't feel anything from it. I was preoccupied. All I could think about was the happy hour my husband and I would go to after the hike. I was hungry, too, but that's not to say I wasn't looking forward to a drink. My favorite things revolved around drinking: wine tastings, beer festivals, and so on. Happy hour was a ten to me. A hike with my favorite person in the world, at a gorgeous waterfall surrounded by an elfin forest, was a five. I thought, *This is great, but I really can't wait for happy hour.* I had learned to *meh* at the wonders of the world, because they couldn't compete with the dopamine manipulation that alcohol brought.

When your brain isn't trained to look for a bigger and better reward, it can find peace and happiness in the here and now. As your neurochemistry rebalances in your alcohol-free brain, your new peaks are suddenly beautiful and yet ordinary, mundane moments. I acutely remember the intensity of this phase. I'd stop, mesmerized by the beauty and wisdom of trees. I'd stare at cloud formations and cry tears of amazement. I'd wake up before sunrises and watch the sky turn pink with starburst energy. I found myself falling in love with classical music and being completely spellbound by pieces that surely I'd heard before and ignored. I'd take in solemn temples and architecture when I traveled, fascinated by human ingenuity and the ability of art to create states of wonder. I was ready to have my breath taken away by the world, waking up after a long slumber and really see it this time.

Wonder is a feeling of surprise mingled with admiration caused by something beautiful, unexpected, unfamiliar, or inexplicable. It stops you in your tracks. Sometimes it's just the realization that you're alive and it's beautiful and even heart wrenching. Wonder and awe can be found everywhere. You merely have to pay attention. Many of my clients experience moments that bring them to tears, awakened to the beauty of the world, not believing how much they had squandered yet feeling so lucky to be awake to it all now. Together, we create anchors for them to remember this feeling and bring themselves back to it anytime the unrest of life gets to them: looking down and counting their five fingers, using a physical object to remind them, or recognizing the power of their breath.

Humans didn't evolve to feel peace or happiness—we evolved to survive. Our brain is always looking for problems. We ruminate on the past or worry about the future. Learning to train your brain to stay in the present and accept the entire breadth of human emotions will teach you how to live with more peace and happiness today.

GRATITUDE

What's the easiest way to tap into this state of wonder and peace? Gratitude. Trust me: When you take an alcohol break with the wrong mindset, it's easy to wallow. I've met plenty of people in the sober world who, when they remove alcohol from their lives, drown in deprivation, frustration, anger, and ultimately helplessness. The focus is on what they're "giving up" instead of recognizing what they're inviting in. By removing alcohol, the world becomes available to you in amazing ways, and the practice of gratitude will help you see that. Students in Become Euphoric™ practice gratitude journaling every day, as part of their Daily Three, which also includes: drink a tall glass of water and state an empowering affirmation.

One way to feel immediately happier—which anyone, anywhere, under any circumstances, can do—is to focus on what you're grateful for. No matter how bad you might think your current situation is, someone, somewhere would do anything to have what you have. *You* get to choose what you focus on. There's always something lacking if lack is what you're looking for. Our brains excel at this. It's how our ancestors survived predators and hostile conditions. Today, we don't have saber-toothed tigers chasing us down. For most of us, our existence isn't as dangerous, but our brain still reacts to problems in the same heightened way.

It's not easy to control your thoughts, so it's up to you to create rituals that uplift you, like a morning gratitude practice. Gratitude is a ritual I practice most days, when I focus on five things I'm grateful for from the previous day. It trains my brain to be on the lookout for blessings and invites more blessings my way. A gratitude practice can even rewire your brain. I look back at some of the emotionally harder times in my life and see how deprived I was of gratitude. When I was twenty-four, I was angry at the world because I didn't have a better job and was jealous of others who seemed to have it all figured out.

Today, I realize I *did* have it all. I had doting parents who helped me financially in college and afterward until I settled on my own. I lived right next to the beach and was able to go for runs along the water. I had a serious boyfriend (Robert, now my husband) who loved me to no end. And while I may have had an entry-level position, I worked at an organization that cared about its employees and had great benefits. In reality, I was blessed, but my relationship with alcohol made it hard to see that. I was stuck in negative feelings, anxiety, and playing out the same old pattern week after week.

And sometimes, the smallest things make you happy. There's something special about enjoying a morning cup of coffee or tea to its fullest. There's something peaceful about laying your head on your pillow and feeling satisfied about your day and the deep slumber you're off to. We'll never be able to control the state of the world and what happens "out there." But you can control what meaning you give to it and what you choose to focus on.

PRESENCE

Being alcohol-free also allows you to be present. Alcohol creates a state of mindlessness because it slows down your neurons, numbs your senses, and makes conscious critical thinking harder. It's no wonder we do and say things while under the influence that are out of alignment with who we want to be. Feeling fully present in the here and now is a tremendous gift. While many parents today use drinking as a way to cope with the challenges of raising children (with stupid marketing slogans like "the most expensive part of having kids is all the wine you have to drink"), there's something to be found by leaning in instead.

One of my clients, Nicole, shared with me how different parenting has become for her since she stopped drinking. Every uncomfortable moment used to be a race to get through, and wine was often the only "solace" she had to deal with the stress of raising little kids. She told me how vastly her relationship with her children has changed, because being alcohol-free allows her to be a fully present parent. She feels more joy, gratitude, and fulfillment by being completely present and aware to the experience, and not numbing or dulling a chunk of her time. Instead of sitting at the playground wishing time would go faster, she feels happy in the moment as she watches her kids play. She's no longer looking outside of herself for comfort; she's found it within. Things can still be hard, but she's learned that the edges aren't so rough when she's not trying to escape them. Her resilience and ability to sit through her emotions and trying times has increased tenfold.

CHAPTER 10

Feel More Joy

ecause alcohol does such a serious number on your brain's neurochemistry, taking a break allows the delicate, natural levels of chemicals that affect your mental health to rebalance. Your serotonin and GABA levels increase, as does your dopamine receptivity. Plus, you stop introducing so many stress hormones into your body. In essence, a break will help clear out your neural pathways, giving you a mental reset. I remember laughing, singing, dancing, and crying in gratitude at the beauty of my life. I laughed so hard a few times, like I hadn't laughed since I was a child. I felt alive. Keep focusing on the benefits, and you'll discover a new way of seeing the world.

I CAN STILL HAVE FUN?

When I start working with clients or leading students through a guided break, there's always a hesitancy in the air. *What if I'm giving up on fun and excitement? What if I run out of things to do? What if I'm boring? What if life is boring?* It's totally valid to feel that way, because alcohol's dopamine manipulation trains your brain to feel that way. I was right there with you thinking that drinking is what made life fun. But it's a myopic viewpoint created when you don't explore what organically gives you joy and excitement. Life is exhilarating. And when you take off the blinders, you start to see it in high definition. One of the greatest epiphanies I get to witness is when clients realize they can have a lot more fun when they don't drink. It's like they're discovering a part of themselves they didn't know existed.

Take Anne, for instance. It was her birthday, and she went on a getaway to the city with her husband and some close friends. While she was nervous about not drinking in such a party atmosphere, she ended up having one of the best birthdays ever. She did it all. Drank mocktails by the pool, went out to nice dinners, talked and laughed with her friends, and woke up at 6:00 a.m. for morning runs in the park. She even felt bad for her friends who went the drinking route and missed out on a lot.

My client Jen went on a camping trip with her boyfriend and couldn't believe what she discovered. She felt so happy, staring up at the stars while sitting by the fire. She felt such freedom not to be worried about alcohol and was connected with her boyfriend in a beautiful moment instead. She was nervous camping wouldn't be as fun without alcohol, yet she'd forgotten for a moment—as we all do—that she lives in a magically abundant universe. Whether you believe in a creator or the infinite wisdom of the universe to expand as it did, we live in a playground of magic. Just look up at the stars one night. Think about white beaches and luscious jungles and snow-capped mountains. You weren't meant to experience any of these natural wonders in a numbed or dulled state.

NEW EXPERIENCES

Seeing life in a new way means you'll also be ready to *experience* life in a new way. And what better way than stepping outside your norm and doing new things? If drinking is your source of fun, you'll have to do some discovery work to find a new version of fun. When I gave up alcohol, I remember doing so many new things. I watched sunrises. I took bike rides along the coast. I did yoga on a paddleboard. I went to writer's groups. I did Zumba. I watched even more sunsets. I went to the symphony, to the botanical gardens, to museums.

Julia Cameron, author of *The Artist's Way*, explains that these dates with yourself, which she terms "artist dates,"[1] are how you can tap into your creativity. Most of us aren't born knowing what our purpose or true calling is, and it's intimidating to figure out. Without knowing it, I was going on all these artist dates, just by being open to new experiences and building my own creativity to find my purpose.

In week 7 of the plan, you're going to dive headfirst into having all kinds of new experiences because, in addition to being fun and a breath of fresh air outside your usual routine, they also help you determine what makes you happy and how you want to spend your time (which could lead to your mission and financial independence). If you have a desire to start a garden or learn how to paint, it's because you're meant to do so. Maybe your purpose in life isn't becoming a landscape artist or a painter, but letting yourself have these experiences may be how your soul calls you toward the direction you're intended to go. After taking the Become Euphoric™ course, my client Caroline turned to new activities that even the best of us would be amazed by, like boxing and learning how to do aerial yoga. All in her midlife—she's a new person.

There may be interests you've long tucked away as ridiculous, like ballroom dancing, tai chi, or photography. Whether these new skills or experiences lead directly to a new passion or just give you more time and space to think and dream, they help you expand your identity. When you feel like you have nothing to do past 5:00 p.m., it's common to feel bored at first, yet boredom is an invitation. Boredom inspires humans to create. Challenge yourself to do something you find interesting but perplexing. Your brain craves the stimulation.

EMBRACING JOY

You are meant to feel good. Well-being is meant to flow through you. Exceptional joy allows divine wisdom and creativity to come through you. When you feel joy, you're in tune with the highest expression of yourself. Living in your zone of joy allows you to be the best version of yourself and uplift the world with your spirit and gifts, making other people feel good too. Shame, guilt, and resentment are soul-eating emotions. If you feel these regularly, which can be inevitable as a drinker, that negative energy will continue to block the positive life you wish for yourself. One secret to living your dream life is feeling great!

Alcohol is a great tool to use when you want to numb the uncomfortable, the boring, the stressful, the sad. But you can't selectively numb the bad and not numb the good as well. Feeling happier isn't a matter of blocking your negative emotions but rather processing them. In week 5, I'll share with you tools you can use to feel and work through all your emotions. When you let your emotions flow and process them in healthier ways, you'll find more states of happiness and joy.

Have you ever heard of the Law of Attraction? It's the concept that your thoughts and overall vibe create your reality.

When you think positively and look for solutions, you create them in your life. When you complain and live in a negative state, you become blind to the opportunities around you. People who always complain aren't going to stumble upon their dream life one day by luck. Or find it when they're feeling low after drinking. No matter how hard I tried to keep it "balanced," drinking always lowered my vibe and made me feel negative the next day. It also prevented me from taking action toward the things I wanted. Changing my relationship with alcohol immediately raised my vibe and state of mind. Life blossomed. The universe started showing me miracles, signs that I was on the right path—little synchronicities like winning free alcohol-free drinks, a free ticket to a personal growth conference, and all-expenses paid trips to Scotland, Costa Rica, and Spain. My friend Chelsea says being alcohol-free allows her to connect deeply to her intuition. When you raise your vibe and energy levels, you attract more goodness and abundance into your life.

LETTING GO OF WHAT
NO LONGER SERVES YOU

If drinking lowers your vibe and dulls your happiness over time, is it worth retaining? I love this mantra from yoga: let go of what no longer serves you. Perhaps drinking served you in the past, but there's nothing wrong with letting it go to invite in who you're supposed to become and grow into. Saying no has such a negative connotation in our society, yet sometimes saying no means saying yes to your truest desires for yourself. You do it all the time in your life, to grow, evolve, and change. Think about what happens when you get married. You are effectually saying no to dating any other man or woman for the rest of your life. However, getting married isn't about the no you're saying to all other dating partners—it's about the yes you're saying to a soulful love that will grow and nourish you as a person and couple.

Life is full of transitions and growing out of old identities. We change our beliefs. We change our lifestyles. I'm not the same person I was at age twenty-five or thirty. Thank god. I've outgrown her. How can you reposition a no in order to see what beautiful blessings will manifest through it?

INSPIRATION AND CREATIVITY

When you let go of what no longer serves you, you create space for something new. The ancient Greeks believed in muses coming to visit writers, poets, and philosophers, to inspire their boldest works and move them beyond their human imaginations. I love the idea of having a channel with something beyond yourself to create beautiful things in this world.

For years, that beautiful channel that calls out creativity was completely blocked for me. I used to write poems and short stories when I was little. I used to journal voraciously. I drew. I danced ballet. And it's incredible to trace the disappearance of those creative outlets. By the time I was in college, and a drinker, I could barely write a page. I've had a handful of ideas for novels over the years but could barely move beyond the first paragraph. I had no discipline. It's easier to drink wine on the couch and watch TV than to write the next great American novel. Why put my heart on the line when I could bury myself in mediocrity and not bother to try?

I didn't know how to show up for myself with tenacity, and I definitely didn't have the vulnerability it takes to write. Writing takes a lot of vulnerability—most writers use what they know from their own life, and many of my experiences were tinged in shame. I didn't want to go there. All I knew was how to numb my thoughts, feelings, and emotions, not how to explore them and develop them. Drinking didn't train me to do that kind of work, to dig deep. It taught me to sit complacently and bury that potential. I could barely even write about my life experiences in a journal, because the backbone of my inner life revolved around letting myself down. Every single year, I'd make a New Year's resolution to write. And each and every year was a disappointment. I almost never felt like writing, so I left it at that. I told myself a story that I didn't enjoy doing hard things. The things that pleased other people, like doing well in work or getting two master's degrees, I could do. But for myself and my big dreams? I didn't show up.

So *poof* went my writing goals, and *poof* went any healthy creative outlet with myself. Because that's what creativity asks of you. You have to open up a channel with your inner guide. You must be willing to be honest and vulnerable. And if you're blocked to greater truths about yourself, it blocks the whole channel. As I mentioned earlier, you can't numb the bad without also numbing the good.

Imagine what happens when you unblock that channel with your creative muse. I felt a cosmic shift, with signs and messages everywhere for me to uncover. The muse told me to create Euphoric. Just two months into my journey, I was in Hawaii when that word started to show up and become relevant for me. A month later, one afternoon I felt a flash of inspiration. I sat down and listened and did more in a single afternoon than I'd ever done as a drinker. I created my brand, my website, my vision and message, and even this very book's structure. I couldn't believe I had all that inside me. I couldn't believe I could tap into it, the source, and create in a way that was impossible for me in a numbed and complacent state. My muse is my intuition, my inner guide. Since then, she's led me to create a lot of things, like programs, retreats, and courses. She's always guiding me, step by step, to live out my potential and manifest the unique gifts I was given.

Creativity is humankind's birthright. It's not just for artsy types. Whether it's refurbishing furniture or baking and selling your own bread, you were meant to be a creator and create things that didn't exist before. But it takes a lot of honesty and overcoming a thick wall of resistance to uncover it. What's the alternative? Sitting on the sidelines of wishes, bitterness, rationalizations, and ultimately despair? That despair may be the reason we're all drinking in the first place. If you find yourself stuck at any time, connect to a bigger question: What do I really want to do in this world? Maybe it's writing a book, launching a business, running for office, or saving the world. You have one life. Use your beautiful mental energy and time on something that fulfills you.

MENTAL TIME AND ENERGY

What surprises women I work with is how much mental time and space they reclaim. Even if the act of drinking only took up 10 percent of their time, suddenly much more is open for new ideas and new activities. And it's not only drinking time you get back. You have to add in the time for the mental gymnastics, the time for not feeling your best, the time for recrimination and guilt, the time for planning and shopping, and the time you're simply hoping the world would speed by faster, because you can't wait for the weekend or until the next drink. Your time increases exponentially when you don't drink. Mornings expand when you're not sleeping off alcohol or sleep deprived.

Your mind isn't preoccupied with shame or regret. Your evenings become intentional as you work on yourself, start new projects, or spend quality time with those you love.

While it's easy to fall into the trap of thinking, *It's too late for me*, or *I've already wasted enough time—what's the point?* The point is huge. Regardless of where you are right now, your timing is perfect. It doesn't matter if you're in your thirties or sixties. It doesn't matter if you've had more than a few Day Ones or if this is the first time you're thinking about a break. It doesn't matter how much time you think you've wasted. It doesn't matter if you think it's too late for you to make a real change and go after what you really want in life. You were meant to be here at this exact time in this exact place and challenge yourself to grow.

One day, you'll look back and see how all the mistakes and regrets have led you to create the life of your dreams. That all the suffering led you to a new perspective, appreciation for life, and sense of empowerment. All your challenges are there for one reason: to turn inward and connect with your soul's purpose. Problems grow you and help you realize what you want most.

Life is short, and you deserve to stop hitting the snooze button on it. You deserve to be fully alive to it instead of sleepwalking through it. You deserve to have healthy self-esteem and confidence. You deserve to love yourself so much that drinking doesn't even cross your mind. You deserve to be happy, healthy, and to evolve to your fullest potential. You certainly don't deserve to be held back by a fermented beverage in a glass. Let's take our power back!

CHAPTER 11

Make Your Relationships Thrive

B *ut everyone around me drinks. How can I possibly navigate my social life without drinking? Plus, I have social anxiety. And it's the glue that makes date night fun.*

Some version of that played on repeat in my head for years. Socializing used to be the bane of my good intentions. I would resolve to take some time off alcohol, only to go to a dinner party that week and cave. I couldn't fathom socializing without alcohol. I was uncomfortable in my own skin. But going alcohol-free not only has given me the confidence to show up as myself out in the world, it also has given me a chance to bond with others on a whole new level.

I'm an introvert. I love reading, going to bed early, and having incredible one-on-one conversations. I need plenty of me time and value my independence. Growing up, I was shy. When I first started drinking as a teenager, alcohol was like a magical elixir that made me talkative, the life of the party, and popular (so I thought). From the start, I picked up a belief that I needed alcohol to be fun and outgoing. It perfectly merged with my teenage insecurities and formed a foundation for my relationship with alcohol into my twenties. Many people are initiated into drinking in their teen years—a time that's rife with insecurities. A lot of us carry these initial associations and bonds with alcohol throughout our adult lives.

Socializing without alcohol is a superpower. Combine it with not worrying about what people think, and you can truly show up as the real you. When you're able to be authentic without a liquid crutch, you'll connect better with others and form stronger bonds than any flimsy connection over multiple rounds. I mean, have you ever died of embarrassment the next day after making a fake new bestie, with promises to visit each other across state? Or was that just me?

I'm going to walk you through exactly how it's possible not only to navigate the world without alcohol but also to strengthen the meaningful connections in your life and attract more incredibly supportive people to your circle. And in week 4 of the plan, I'll make sure you know exactly how to have a great time at the party and let go of your FOMO (fear of missing out) by giving you the mindset tool you need to appreciate each social occasion without alcohol. Even though I thought alcohol got me out of my shell, it really made me more insecure, lonely, and disengaged from others. My objections from the start of the chapter were nothing more than self-limiting beliefs. Meaningful connections in your life are not dependent on the contents of your glass.

WHAT ABOUT MY PARTNER?

This question always comes up with my partnered clients. Often, we share drinking with the people who are close in our lives, most commonly with our partners. It's a regular part of the relationship. How do you make changes without turning it all upside down?

I met my husband when I was twenty-three years old. Those were my "wild" years. I was still partying hard in graduate school and was deeply entrenched in the habits I'd picked up boozing through college. Thankfully, settling down to a healthy adult relationship helped change my focus from the bar scene to building a life together—complete with trips to IKEA, runs along the boardwalk, and a juicing diet craze. And, yes, alcohol still. Even as "responsible adults," our drinking life together was filled with trips to wineries across the border, beers by the pool, brewery visits, and a bottle of wine with Netflix. Drinking was a pastime for date night, movie night, game night, Sunday night—you name it.

What happens when you shake that up?

You invite in a pause, a reevaluation, and a chance to get to know each other in an entirely new way. My first year alcohol-free was a brand-new year for me and my husband. We had to learn to connect with each other all over again. And today, I can say with 100 percent certainty that we are closer in values, more deeply bonded, and spend way more quality time together than ever before.

When I was drinking, I wasn't being completely honest with him, because I was numbing the parts of me I didn't like. Learning to embrace who I am helped free me to then show that person to the people I really love. I opened up, became vulnerable, and started painting a vision that was so much bigger than our previous reality.

Exploring an alcohol-free life is all about personal growth. When you redevelop a relationship with yourself and your inner guide, you process your own needs and therefore become a better partner and are able to devote the time and presence to nurture your relationship. Though I'm busier than ever, my husband and I have more quality time together, because no time is made blurry with alcohol. We moved some of our "date" nights outside and trained for a half-marathon together. We love to play board games together—even those twelve-round legacy games that take months. We dream together. Emotionally, I've learned not to bottle up my insecurities or frustrations—I allow myself to be who I am and share my concerns or fears. I feel like I finally see him instead of seeing past him. I'm incredibly lucky to have a partner who has watched me grow and is excited by my transformation instead of threatened by it.

It's not always like that right away, and that's okay. Remember that any lifestyle change, even a positive one, takes getting used to. For example, if your husband's alarm clock wakes you every morning at 5:00 a.m. so he can go for a run, you might be annoyed about your disrupted sleep. Even though he's doing something good for himself, it's hard to understand when you're not doing it too. Did my husband completely understand what I was going through? No, not at first. But I was open to making changes in myself first, believing that working on myself was worth it and would eventually strengthen our marriage. Here are some things to keep in mind while going through the adjustment.

Your dearest loved ones want you to be happy, but they might not understand your decision and may fear that you'll drift away. That's entirely normal. Change brings up fear in other people that they'll lose you, or you'll outgrow them. You can use this opportunity to talk and learn about what your partner needs.

You also don't need your partner onboard for you to make positive lifestyle changes. For instance, if you wanted to go back to graduate school, would you complain that it's impossible unless your partner does it with you? Be codependent no more. You're allowed to let go of what no longer serves you and grow regardless of whether your partner is game. Your journey is your journey. Don't try to change them and their behavior. The best thing you can do is work on yourself and become a radiant inspiration for other people. You never know what you may inspire, but people need their own autonomy to change.

As you're exploring a new way of living, don't forget about them! Actively find new ways to spend quality time together. Get creative. Run a race, learn a new hobby together, and make sure you have a mocktail you love for patio time or game nights. You can still spend time together decompressing over drinks. What's in your glass isn't what keeps you and your partner bonded.

DATING ALCOHOL-FREE

I get it. When you're dating, meeting up for drinks is usually the first date. It's been a hot minute since I've been on the dating scene, but back in the day, there was no way I would put myself out there without a drink in hand. Drinking is supposed to smooth away the awkward edges, right? Plus, isn't it expected? But when you drink to deal with nerves or bond with someone, you aren't connecting in an authentic way. Haven't you ever initiated a "thing" at a party while under the influence, only to realize later that you have nothing in common with that person? Alcohol shuts down your intuition and makes it hard to discern if you truly like someone. Alcohol makes the choice for you. I've fallen into plenty of relationships because "drinking me" thought it was a good match (in other words, the guy was hot), and inertia kept me in a relationship I shouldn't have been in. When you use the artificial stimulation of a drink to bond, you get an artificial outcome.

My married lifestyle doesn't give me an opportunity to explore these dynamics in real life, but I have plenty of single girlfriends who tell me about their alcohol-free dating adventures. Here's the ugly: Some people will feel uncomfortable with the idea that you don't drink. You know that saying, "It's them, not you"? That's what's at play here. People are uncomfortable with the idea of you not drinking if they don't like how you are holding up a mirror to their own behavior. If someone is turned off by the idea of you not drinking, it's a huge blessing in disguise. It's highly likely they've got their own complicated thing going on with alcohol or are myopic about the way things have to be. You're doing yourself a favor by weeding out potential partners who are threatened by you living your best life, have their own complicated relationship with alcohol, or are locked into their own limiting stories.

While alcohol-free dating can be awkward initially, Amanda, my friend in Texas, has a no-nonsense approach. Either include your alcohol-free status in your dating profile, along with "dog lover" and "avid hiker," or ask the person to go on a creative first date. Shake up the bar routine and ask your potential date to do something fun instead. Try hiking, grabbing coffee or boba, or going bowling. If they're not into it, they're probably not interested in truly getting to know you. Feeling a little vulnerable together can help you get to know a deeper side of them and weed out the emotionally intelligent men (or ladies) from the jerks. Remember that *you* choose what you put into your body. Would you let someone give you crap about eating vegetarian or gluten-free? Don't let someone do the same about what you choose to drink or not drink.

When you're focused on living your life, feeling amazing, having the mental space to go after your dreams, and truly taking care of yourself, you become a magnet of energy that attracts other high-vibe people into your life. When you ditch alcohol, you create space for much better things, so start to think about the same thing happening in your dating life. Some of the most successful, goal-getting, unstoppable figures we admire out there are alcohol-free. Many entrepreneurs and athletes don't drink because they want to optimize their life, not detract from it.

Today, I'm a magnet for high-vibe women and men who either don't drink or drink so occasionally that alcohol is irrelevant in their lives. While you may think I find these people because of what I do, I find them in the unlikeliest places in my life. Like attracts like, so envision yourself attracting the upgraded, emotionally intelligent, amazing man (or woman) who matches your new vibe.

ADVANTAGES TO REMEMBER WHILE DATING ALCOHOL-FREE

- You can determine whether you like someone without alcohol goggles
- You bond more authentically and deeply
- You can separate the tools from the real deals
- You attract a better partner

MAKING NEW FRIENDS

One of my longtime friends is a natural at making friends and keeping up with them. She throws parties and events and has a big circle of people whom she cares about. I used to compare myself to her, and it made me feel woefully socially inept. After college, many of my good girlfriends spread out to other cities, as did I. In my twenties, living in a new town, I was stumped. How the hell do you make adult friends?

If I can figure this one out, without drinking, so can you. It's a fear-based belief that's telling you that you're giving up your social life when you ditch alcohol. In reality, you're positioning yourself to dramatically increase it.

Scientists say humans are prone to addictive behaviors when they're isolated and lonely.[1] What's lonelier than pretending everything is fine when it's not? Or fake friends forged over boozy conversation that you can't remember the next day? Alcohol disconnects you from others, so much so that when you go alcohol-free, you're ready for real connection. You no longer want to fake it or bond over small talk. You start to look for authentic connections with growth-oriented seekers who honor your new life.

You'll get excited to seek out your empowering lifestyle reflected in other badass women and men. The friends I've made in the alcohol-free community have completely transformed my life. It's a space designed for love and support, and it's ever growing with enthusiasm. And these spaces are popping up everywhere! I'm talking about mocktail bars, alcohol-free parties and raves, and tons of social meetups and community groups.

A few months into my exploration, I was so psyched about my new lifestyle and wanted to meet other people who could relate (and jump up and down with me). It's like a secret discovery you can't wait to share with others who are in on it too. I went to a women's alcohol-free brunch meetup, and I was a little nervous I wouldn't fit in. Would this be like an AA meeting over pancakes? The organizer of the event, Danielle, and

I started sharing our stories and views on alcohol-free life. We had much in common. A few years earlier, I'd been baffled by people who made adult friends. Now, I found myself easily and naturally hanging out and deepening our friendship. Today, she is one of my closest friends, and we have a podcast together, all about how amazing alcohol-free life is. (Add *Euphoric the Podcast* to your library today!) Even our respective partners are great friends.

Danielle is such a guidepost for me, and I regularly seek her advice. I'm grateful this incredible friendship all started because my inner voice was telling me I needed more connection, and I was brave enough to listen and put myself out there. Along with our other friend Angela, Danielle and I also host San Diego's MindBar, a downtown mocktail party and intention-setting evening for hip women who want a vibrant social life without a side of hangovers. After each social hour with these women, I feel so lit up and abuzz, alcohol can't even compare. We talk about real things and challenge ourselves to live unapologetically in all areas of our lives.

There's a new social club that revolves around #women-empoweringwomen alcohol-free. If nothing exists yet in your city, why not create it? My client Lacey found herself living in a new city with few friends. Instead of feeling defeated, she chose to start her own alcohol-free community and made several close friends in a matter of weeks. I can't help but feel so inspired by the ripple effects we can create when we choose to show up fully and lead the women standing with us. While introverted me over here still needs my solitude, still isn't a fan of networking events, and still hates to pick up my phone, I get to be intentional about the connections I do form in my life and go to things like brunch and personal growth retreats, or out for mocktails with other incredible women. I also seek out masterminds and sister circles with women all over the world. The people I surround myself with are growth-oriented and inspire me to reach for my biggest goals. Community in your life doesn't need to come with a side of hangover and regret. In week 4 of the program, I'll give you the full scoop on finding the alcohol-free dreamers who live in your vicinity and all over the world.

NAVIGATING WITH YOUR FRIENDS AND FAMILY

I have something to tell you: Your dearest friends and family love you for who you are. Full stop. They don't love you because of what you drink or who you become when your brain is hijacked by alcohol. When you use an extended break from alcohol to become more intentional about your life, you can also become more intentional about the relationships you have with the loved ones currently in your life. The process might have some hiccups, but those hiccups are solvable.

The biggest lie I told myself about alcohol was that it made me more comfortable in my skin. I learned this lesson hard and fast as an introverted teen and kept up this limiting story throughout my twenties. It pains me to say this, but hanging out with my closest friends and family without drinking made me incredibly nervous. While I didn't do much deep introspection into the why back then, today I realize I was afraid that I wasn't good enough as myself—that I wasn't likeable, interesting, or fun. Alcohol was like a flimsy glue I used to try to pull it all together. A fake veneer.

And I'm not alone in those thoughts. Our society teaches us that socializing goes hand in hand with alcohol. It's the quick solution to awkwardness and social anxiety. If you've been drinking since high school, have you ever learned how to socialize without it? As with any skill, it's not something you're born with. You have to practice! In week 4, we'll go over my favorite tips on how to rock a party, engage meaningfully in conversations, and make sure your mindset is ready to embrace an incredible social life—plus tips on what to say to own your choice proudly.

When I removed alcohol from the equation when hanging out with my friends, slowly but surely, I started to feel safe just being myself. I started talking about things that mattered to me—my fears, my vulnerabilities, and my biggest dreams. I no longer used alcohol to hide and with practice built up confidence and felt comfortable in my own skin, instead of looking for something outside of me to give me a false sense of comfort. And my friends appreciated it. I would say we are much closer today than ever before. Pretending everything is okay and that you have your life together (and not letting anyone in) is the very thing that disallows us to connect authentically with others.

Even sharing your feelings toward alcohol and the shifts you're having during your break can be the piece of vulnerability that your friendships need to thrive. When I was finally honest about my relationship with alcohol, I was calling it how it is, and you'll be surprised at how many of your friends feel the same sentiment. (Think you're the only one who hates how you feel the morning after drinking?)

That doesn't mean it will be easy! Like attracts like, right? So, it's probably no coincidence that most of your friends are drinkers too. Remember how most humans react toward change: It's scary. One, you are holding up a mirror to your friend's behavior—behavior he or she might feel insecure about. Two, when you change, people often fear they will lose you and that you will outgrow them. Those are legitimate fears. With time, patience, grace, and adjustment, the people who are meant to be in your life to support and cheer you on will eventually rise to the occasion, and you can work through those issues together. The people who can't might slowly fall off the radar. Set boundaries for anyone who doesn't want the best for you. Your social life will change, but often in a really good way. Invite in more honest conversation, spend time doing new things, and attract high-vibe people into your life. You might start to choose to hang out with people who uplift you more than the people who bring you down. Isn't that the most beautiful thing about being an adult? You get to choose.

Most of the time, we worry about what other people will think. We hardly stop and ask ourselves if we admire and aspire to the lifestyle of the person whose opinion matters so much. This is where people like your coworkers, in-laws, and random acquaintances sometimes land. (Dealing with your family, whom you don't get to choose, might be more complicated.) If you don't want their life, why do you care what they think? How does their opinion matter in creating the life you do want? Does choosing to focus your energy on them and what they think let you feel happy and free?

After your incredible transformation, I want you to view the world through a new lens, as an observer of human psychology. When friends, family, or random acquaintances don't respond well to your choice not to drink, it provides insight into their own personal issues. And you are growing your emotional resilience to handle their reactions. If you stay small and stuck for others, you'll resent that choice and those people in your life. Love people for who and where they are, but let yourself break free from a limiting pattern, and you'll live without regrets.

CHAPTER 12

Being Alcohol-Free Makes You Brave

COMFORT VERSUS FULFILLMENT

If you're starting to feel expansive and asking yourself, *Who could I be if I didn't hold myself back in this way?* that's your intuition guiding you toward possibility. One of my clients, Amanda, had a quick answer: a CEO. She's on fire as a nondrinker, improving in every area of her life and getting closer to her dream job. She's experienced the physical benefits and energy levels and has a new obsession with hot yoga. She's gone through the redevelopment of positive beliefs about herself with a renewed sense of confidence and pride. And there's also the beautiful aftermath of pushing herself outside her comfort zone on a regular basis. She's going for what she really wants.

Simply put, being alcohol-free makes you brave.

As a drinker, I hung out way too long and way too often in my comfort zone. When I felt uncomfortable or tired or stressed or bored, I retreated to a familiar space where I could shut down for a while. Reaching for a drink whenever I wanted to achieve a state I didn't believe I was capable of reaching on my own, I did little to solve or relieve the problems or feelings that drew me there in the first place. Although I had a handful of comfort-zone behaviors (and ones I still work through), drinking was the go-to behavior, and it's probably one of the most common, unhealthy coping mechanisms out there. And it's not as though healthy coping skills are something we're taught in school.

You know the story: Work is crazy stressful, but by 7:00 p.m., with a glass of wine in your hand, you hardly care, because you can just turn off the nagging thoughts and unresolved to-dos. However, you're not solving the issues that stressed you or truly relaxing your body to better handle future stress. All you're doing is numbing your thoughts and compounding your inability to handle situations proactively when you wake up (yes, feeling lousy).

You can see this play out with all kinds of limiting behaviors. It could be sitting on the couch and gorging on food, getting so full you can't pay attention to your monkey mind. Or compulsively checking your phone and going on social media, attempts to be constantly distracted. Binge-watching TV or online shopping. Even the cult of busyness that many of us fall into, so we never slow down and deal with our inner lives. Now, I'm not talking about treats or vilifying TV. I'm talking about the compulsion to escape.

These behaviors ensure that you can distract or numb your thoughts and emotions away. Of course, that's not the motivation in the moment. All you know is that you feel a little off, and while anyone knows that mindlessly scrolling social media for hours doesn't make you feel happy, your comfort zone still gets a lot of time and space because it feels safe and easy and gets you out of your own head for a while.

But it gets pretty dark and twisted when you let what's easy in the moment define your life's path. Because comfort is not the same thing as happiness. And comfort is often standing in your way of fulfillment. Even though my comfort zone of drinking only gave me *false* security, I protected it because I didn't know what was outside my comfort zone. Drinking was painful and unfulfilling, yet making a change seemed way too scary, too unknown, and even extreme. I always regretted drinking. I didn't look forward to social drinking occasions, because I didn't completely trust myself. *Oh great, another opportunity for me to drink more than I want to, hate myself afterward, and feel incredibly shitty for a few days.* What do they call insanity? Doing the same thing over and over again and expecting different results. And it's excruciatingly hard to make any changes, because we're constantly bombarded with the message of the healthy, successful woman who has it all. She wakes up early, goes to the gym, smashes it at her job, goes out with friends for happy hour, and wakes up and does it all over again. One thing doesn't fit with the others.

Fear of change may tell you to stay in your comfort zone or to stay in your status quo. But you have to ask yourself, *What do you really want out of life?* Comfort or fulfillment? A quick fix or true happiness? Most things you want in life are outside your comfort zone. I know ignoring that little voice and staying with the status quo seems So. Much. Easier. After all, change implies risk. Change could even mean failure. Humans resist change because we fear the unknown future and worry it will be worse than where we find ourselves today. At least we know the shape and feel of what we're in today. But familiar and safe? That's the stuff of long-term life regrets, and when you ignore that inner voice, the more unhappy and disappointed in your life you'll be.

And while the voice of comfort and ultimately fear might want you to stay exactly where you are, if you get really quiet, you'll hear an even truer voice: The voice that tells you when you're living life out of alignment with your deeper values and your bigger purpose. The voice of faith over fear. The voice that believes in you. The voice that knows you have infinite potential.

TRAIN YOURSELF TO BE BRAVE

When you smash your self-limiting beliefs—which we discussed in chapter 6 and will further explore in week 1 of the eight-week plan—you awaken your courage. Living a stuck and stagnant life gives you all kinds of reasons to believe you're incapable of going after what you want. But when you take a break and start doing the mindset work, you become confident in your abilities. You become brave and courageous. Instead of quelling your own uniqueness to fit in and live by the expectations of the society around you, you stop elevating other people's opinions over your own well-being.

It takes a lot of courage to stand up for your well-being and happiness when everyone around you is drinking. Breaking free from the status quo means you become an outlier. A wolf among sheep. Don't worry—there are many other wolves around you, waiting to lift you up, empower you, and give you a new sense of belonging when the old sense of belonging doesn't work anymore. Every conversation you have makes you braver and braver. What you're doing isn't just new, it's radical. The bravery you get from not drinking and taking a stand for an alcohol-free life—in a world obsessed with rosé—gives you the courage to go for even bigger and scarier things.

Having the bravery to stand up to a social norm and prioritize yourself over fitting in is often the most liberating experience for my clients. At first, Emma was worried about not drinking at networking events and around her friends, but then she accessed her inner rebel. Today, instead of worrying about fitting in, she's created a ripple effect and inspired her friends.

Living a courageous life isn't about a life absent fear. Fear never completely goes away, because once you overcome one thing, there's a new challenge to overcome. The secret to living a courageous life is about feeling the fear and moving forward anyway. Going alcohol-free trains you to feel the fear and do the scary thing anyway—and to be rewarded with the most amazing miracles on the other side. Telling people builds courage. Ordering a mocktail builds courage. Inviting your friends out for a hike instead of the usual cocktails builds courage. Then, you start using that courage to pursue the things you really want to do, be, and have.

When you commit to showing up and not numbing out, you create a new life. When you commit to listening to your intuition and never being dishonest with yourself again, you create a new way of being. I used to believe it was painful to desire something that seemed unattainable, that it was too scary to let yourself desire something so different from what your current level of courage and strength would allow you to do. But in reality, it's far more painful to settle for mediocrity and let the feelings of wasted potential eat away at you, as you throw out excuse after excuse for why you can't, why you shouldn't, or why it's impossible.

It's not easy to chase your dreams. It can welcome in criticism, skepticism, and judgment. But what's the alternative? Not even trying and living a life full of regrets? Critical of other people because you're jealous and you yourself aren't going for it? No way—never again. I've already lived that life. Being awake to your biggest dreams can feel scary, but it's also what makes you feel alive and builds your resiliency. All that matters is that you show up, imperfectly. You'll gain courage, pride, confidence, patience, love, fulfillment, and ultimately grow spiritually.

CHAPTER 13

Live Up to Your Fullest Potential

BE NORMAL OR BE EXCEPTIONAL

So, do I have to quit drinking forever? That's a loaded question. Personally, I don't use the word *forever*, or even the word *quit*. I'm a nondrinker. Just like I'm a nonsmoker. And a non-streetcar racer. It's my identity, and I don't feel limited by what I don't do, but rather freer for it because of what it allows me to be, do, and have in this lifetime. Wherever you arrive is perfectly okay. But know that you won't arrive overnight. It takes time for your thinking to evolve, so give yourself a chance to let things unfold.

When I was going through this transition, I was falling in love with my new alcohol-free life, but it wasn't easy to embrace the idea of never drinking again. I thought, maybe, just maybe, I'd revisit this drinking thing in a few more months or a year. You know, be someone who drinks only occasionally, like at special events. Would it be possible? Possible, sure, but it takes crazy, Jedi-level mastery to truly moderate and drink occasionally. So why even go there? I thought long and hard about it and realized that if I ever went back to alcohol, I'd be doing it out of my desire to fit in and be "normal."

If you invest all your energy into trying to be "normal," you completely miss the mark for being exceptional. Normal is average, boring, mediocre. We don't love the people we love dearly because of how "normal" they are—we love them because of how unique and special they are. You might value your partner's sense of humor, ambition, or positivity. You might admire your best friend's creativity, bravery, or humility. Their uniqueness is precisely why you love them.

In the quest to be "normal" and fit in, we lose our intrinsic selves—the very essence that makes you you, that makes you truly extraordinary, even exceptional. For far too long, I lived my life striving to be accepted and normal, and letting other peoples' opinions determine my worth. I already knew what this life felt like. I knew exactly what it felt like to be a drinker. What I didn't know was what I was capable of as a nondrinker. I didn't know what I was capable of without a toxin holding me back. Did I want to push the envelope of my potential or cling dearly to mediocrity and fitting in? The choice was easy.

At the end of the eight-week plan, I'll guide you through next steps and options, because you have full autonomy to make any choices in your life. But when you feel confused or doubtful, try to examine your reasons for wanting to go back to drinking. With some scrutiny and self-love, you might find your deeper wisdom again showing you the answer. Pushing myself out of my comfort zone was the best thing I've ever done for myself, yet there will always be a fear-based reason tugging you to go back to alcohol. You have to decide—will you choose faith over fear? Expansion over contraction? Showing up 100 percent over phoning it in?

CHOOSING YOUR DREAMS

Brian Tracy shares a brilliant analogy in his book *No Excuses!: The Power of Self-Discipline.* We all live on Someday Isle. Someday Isle is full of wishes: Someday I'll write a book. Someday I'll have financial independence. Someday I'll freely travel the world. Someday I'll have my own business and make an impact. Until I changed my relationship with alcohol, it never even dawned on me that I could do anything about those goals in the present moment. I had no idea where or how to start. If a genie had magically appeared, I would have been ready with my wishes, but to actually work on them in the present? That was a foreign concept to me.

Hope is not a strategy. A dream will never manifest itself if you don't work on it. It takes discipline, perseverance, and motivation to achieve your goals. But alcohol teaches us to do what's easy in the moment instead of what brings long-term fulfillment. Every time I chose passive, dopamine-manipulating alcohol over experiencing my feelings or creating my own joy, I was taking the easy way out. I didn't learn to feel my feelings, process them, or create fun for myself outside of a drink. Compounded with the shame, loss of self-esteem, self-doubt, and anxiety about drinking, it was too much to look ahead and build the life of my dreams. I didn't have looking-ahead skills. Instead, I was chasing momentary relief and passive gratification.

When I stopped drinking, something inside me shifted monumentally. It was a huge wake-up call that I already had everything inside of me to achieve my "someday" goals. I remember sitting in the park one afternoon and sketching out my biggest goals coming to life. I had never allowed myself to dream so audaciously. I started visualizing who I wanted to be in this world. I stopped waiting for my dream life to fall into my lap. And since that day, I've been on a trajectory to fulfill those dreams.

My someday dreams took years to fulfill (and now I have new and bigger ones). It's easy to get discouraged and disappointed that they aren't happening fast enough. We love overnight fixes and quick wins. You might even feel discouraged that changing your relationship with alcohol has taken so long. But here's what you need to remember: the time will pass by either way. Five years from now, you can be certain of one thing: five years will have passed. So who cares if it takes five years to go after your dream? Who cares if it takes five years to grow into the person you want to be? Who cares if it takes five years to grow your side hustle and leave your day job? It took me four years to get this book into your hands. Imagine if I'd given up after one year because it wasn't happening fast enough? Your someday dreams will take time to manifest. But the time will pass by either way, and you may as well use it striving toward something that fulfills your soul. Bill Gates is famous for saying, "Most people overestimate what they can do in one year and underestimate what they can do in ten years."[1]

You can choose to see a long road ahead and get discouraged trying to figure out the "how." Or you can continue to dream up what you really want, access your deeper why, and take each baby step that the universe presents to you. My dream started with the tiniest baby step, in building my website. I listened to that call, and then the universe showed me the next baby step to take, and the next one after that. I never gave up, and I rested along the way.

Today, I can't believe the lifestyle I have because I listened to that call. I do what I love for a living. I make money by helping others let go of what no longer serves them and step into their bigger dreams. I can work from any destination in the world. I frequently travel to places like St. Thomas, Puerto Vallarta, and Tulum. I'm friends with my heroes. I get to share my story and message in articles, on podcasts, and on stages. I get plant-based meals delivered to my doorstep. I learn from masters and regularly go to conferences, masterminds, and retreats. I'm growing and scaling the business of my dreams. I am constantly growing and, because of that, impact other people's lives. You can't give if you don't grow. I hear from women all the time who say I've helped them radically change their life: *I wrote and published a book! I love my body. I love myself. I love my life!*

A few years ago, my current life was all a pipe dream. But when I changed one fundamental part of my identity, it opened the floodgates to change my entire definition of self. Believe in where you're going. Let your faith spill over into every area of your life. I get so excited to see clients reach this phase, because there's a spark in their eyes and a determination to chase dreams they long ago shelved.

One client, Christie, launched a spiritual gifts business and spends her weekends creating art that she sells instead of mopping up the mess of a night out. Tiffany wrote a book about women empowering women and building the economy in her local community. Ann started drawing outside again. Sara grew her business by 50 percent and is scaling to hit $1 million in revenue. Lindsay started an Etsy shop for her macramé art. Laura got certified as a coach and started her own coaching business. Erin went back to school to become a therapist. Lacey launched her own holistic community for women. Andrew took on a leadership role in his company. Patrick moved halfway across the world and travels to far-out destinations to windsurf. Sarah built a course positioning her as an expert in her field. Cara is planning her move to Europe. Julie went back to her childhood dream of becoming a writer and is writing her first book.

This is why I do what I do. This is what fuels me. I don't care about the beverage that's in your glass. I care that you're awake to your life. The transformation I had and get to witness with my community is beyond any surface-level changes. Transform your relationship with alcohol, and it will change your entire life.

It feels so good to follow your own North Star, and I can tell you with 100 percent certainty that none of this would have happened when I still thought the highlight of the week was a bottle of wine. Because a bottle of wine ends with nothing. No growth or development. No help attaining your life goals. And while it gives nothing, it erodes so much more. What do we have to show for all that alcohol consumed?

BE THE STAR OF YOUR OWN LIFE

One of my favorite quotes by Theodore Roosevelt, from his "The Man in the Arena" speech reminds me that we have two choices in life—either be in the arena or sit on the sidelines:

> The credit belongs to the man who is actually in the arena, whose face is marred by dust and sweat and blood; who strives valiantly; who errs, who comes short again and again, because there is no effort without error and shortcoming [. . .] who at the best knows in the end the triumph of high achievement, and who at the worst, if he fails, at least fails while daring greatly.[2]

You weren't meant to live your life sitting on the sidelines of the arena. You were meant to dare greatly. There is no one more important than you in your life. This isn't just about alcohol. It's about you stepping into the arena and no longer hiding in the audience. I'm done playing small in my life and letting a beverage (of all things!) dictate how I feel about myself. I don't stare wistfully or jealously from the sidelines of my own life anymore. I work hard to be the star in it. And you deserve to be the star in yours too.

Together, we're going to work on changing your habits, yes, but even more so your patterns of thinking, your subconscious beliefs, how you respond to the world, your inner dialogue, your sense of self-love. The idea that I have only one life to live and that I better be the star in it is my deeper why and can rattle me out of the deepest status quo. You, my dear reader, are a star. Cherish it.

If you think drinking might be holding you back, then it already is. This is serious stuff, but trust me, an approach to the alcohol-free life doesn't have to be. It's not all or nothing, and in part III, it's time to take what you've learned and apply it with healthy curiosity to try something new. If you're ready to see what you're capable of when you don't hold yourself back, then let's go!

PART III

Your Eight-Week
Plan to Ditch Alcohol
and Gain a Happier,
More Confident You

Y ou did it! You finished parts I and II of this book. To me, you're already super committed and a star. Not everyone gets this far. You're not afraid to go deep, challenge cultural assumptions, and uncover who you are authentically and what really makes you happy. As I've mentioned, at the end of the day, this isn't about a fermented beverage: it's about discovering who you really are, what you honestly need, and what you truly desire to be, do, and have in this one lifetime. These next eight weeks will focus on those three big challenges and help you experiment with a lifestyle that brings out the best in you and allows you to follow your North Star. Only you get to decide what kind of person you want to continue to grow into.

The beauty of this process is that you don't have to decide to quit drinking forever. In fact, I recommend not to, at first. Any time you drink too much, have horrible sleep, or a headache the next day will cause you to chastise yourself: "Never again!" We've all been there. Many women get stuck in this loop, as I was for many years. They vow on Monday morning that they'll quit drinking. Then, by Thursday or Friday night, the cravings or social events are back, and the Monday morning vows seem like crazy talk. *What the hell was I thinking? I'll start that next week. I'm not going to quit drinking today.* And the desire to live alcohol-free continues to get pushed off, week after week after week. Do you know what this sounds like to me? Waking up on Monday morning vowing to get married the next day without even meeting the guy! And when you get cold feet, which is normal, you back down. Of course you did, because you didn't even allow yourself to go on the first date!

You don't have to decide about forever today. "Never again!" is something said out of desperation and not true confidence or preference. You'll never get to experience the joys of living and breathing alcohol-free when you're stuck in this I-should-quit-wait-I-can't-quit shouting match in your head. Take marriage off the table and commit to going on the first date.

The first date is your eight-week plan to take a guided break from alcohol and discover your intrinsic self. Eight weeks, or roughly two months, allows you to break the habit, fully experience living in a new way, and rekindle your passions and purpose. If you don't like it, you can go back to drinking when the break ends. But until you take a guided break, you'll never know which way of being you prefer, which lifestyle makes you happier. This is an experiment, and the end result is getting to know yourself better. It's fifty-six days, and I know you can do it. I believe in you!

WHAT TO EXPECT

Tomorrow will be your first day alcohol-free and the first day of the plan—your week 1, day 1. How exciting! The plan lasts eight weeks or fifty-six days of being alcohol-free and focusing on your personal growth. When it's over, you get to decide how to move forward. Each week has lessons for you to read, action steps for you to follow, and journaling homework for you to complete, so you can delve deep. Feel free to read each week's plan at the beginning of the week or space it out to read a section each day. As you continue to learn new things, know this: Your brain is neuroplastic, meaning that as you make new mental connections and associations, you'll be building new neural pathways in your brain. As you let go of beliefs and ideas that no longer serve you, you'll be pruning neural pathways. You have the power to change your brain.

So you can get the best out of this plan, here are some things to keep in mind:

- Commit to doing the plan 100 percent. Decision fatigue is real. Making fifty-six decisions each day is a game of willpower and can cause burnout fast. Commit to the whole thing now and go for it. But if you do slip and drink, don't throw in the towel. Just consider it a blip and keep going! Don't beat yourself up either. It happens. Instead, use it as a learning experience to understand what triggers you. Who you are is defined by the next decision you make, not the previous one. So, get up and keep going.
- Take a photo of yourself and label it "Day Zero."
- Stay positive and curious. This isn't about deprivation. You're exploring yourself and expanding and learning what it feels like to be fully alive. Each new feeling and emotion you go through helps give you a new insight that you can learn from. As you learn, you grow. As you grow, you evolve. If you think this will be hard, it will be. If you experience it with curiosity and an open mind, you'll be blessed in ways you can't imagine.
- Each day in the course, Become Euphoric™, I ask clients to write down three things they're grateful for. It helps attune them to the blessings of this experience and get into a great mindset. No matter who you are or what your life circumstance looks like,

you can find something to be grateful for. Keeping a gratitude journal while you go through the plan will help transform your mindset.

- Drink a tall glass of water first thing every morning. Hydration is really important in healing, especially to cleanse the body of any residual effects of alcohol.

- And last, don't wait to get started. You picked up this book for a reason. Don't wait to do this section *after* the big vacation, wedding, or Mom's birthday party. An event will always be on the horizon. One of my biggest regrets is not starting earlier because I was paralyzed by some event I was convinced required me to drink. Looking back, none of those drinking occasions were worth pressing pause on my personal growth. In weeks 4 and 7, I'll walk you through socializing, vacations, and not feeling like you're missing out. You don't have to hide out for the next eight weeks either. I want you to socialize. While it might feel nerve-racking, you'll never know what muscles you'll build, connections you'll make, and epiphanies you'll have unless you get out there and socialize as the real you.

JOURNALING HOMEWORK

At the end of each week, you'll complete journal reflections or an exercise to tap into your own experiences, feelings, and thoughts. While it's easy to skim through these and think them in your head, don't merely think—write down your thoughts. Studies have proven that we're able to tap into deeper parts of our subconscious when we write things down.[1] Journaling is also proven to improve your mental health and a way to build a solid connection with your intuition.[2] As writer Joan Didion put it, "I don't know what I think until I write it down."[3]

YOUR JOURNALING HOMEWORK

Let's get started on your first journaling assignment. This pre-homework before we begin the plan is meant to help uncover your deeper why. Take out your journal and answer the following questions:

- Why did you pick up this book?
- Why do you want to drink less or not at all? What negative effects about alcohol do you absolutely hate (hangovers, poor sleep, letting yourself down, feeling unhealthy, worrying about it, etc.)? Get specific and try to think of at least ten reasons.
- Who do you hope to become in the process?
- Why is it important to you that you live healthier, be more intentional, and connect with yourself?

Examine and Dismantle Limiting Beliefs

TRUST YOUR INNER GUIDE

Have you ever made a decision that seemingly came out of nowhere? Maybe you had a strong urge to move to another city, take a trip, or leave a company, and you trusted this intuition. And years later, you realize that if you hadn't acted, you wouldn't have received an amazing blessing in your life. Maybe you wouldn't have the life you have today if it weren't for that one decision.

This is the power of your intuition, or the ability to know what the next right step is without conscious, logical reasoning. Your eight-week challenge to ditch alcohol is all about getting back in touch with your intuitive self, or inner guide. It's the wise voice inside you that knows you were made for more. Alcohol fuzzes up your channel to your inner guide. So, we're going to learn how to get back in touch with it, through introspection.

At first you might feel a lot of resistance and fear. This is normal. The opposite of your inner guide, your ego, doesn't want you to change. It doesn't want you to leave the known for the unknown. But author Steven Pressfield gives us this rule of thumb: "The more important a call or action is to our soul's evolution, the more resistance we will feel toward pursuing it."[1] Meaning that feeling resistance right now is a sign that you've got some major breakthroughs coming that probably will change the trajectory of your life—in a good way, of course.

Before we start, I want to say something, loud and clear: there's nothing wrong with you. In the first half of the book, I included as many facts and figures as I could to demonstrate that having a complicated relationship with alcohol is the most common experience a drinker faces. Alcohol is probably one of the most typical coping mechanisms. But just because you or your drinking are not a "problem" doesn't mean that drinking has been helping you go where you want to get in life. And because you're a dreamer and a doer, I know you want to go far, even if that's not something you've admitted to yourself before. You'll never reach that beautiful place if you keep on hanging out in your comfort zone. Drinking alcohol isn't wrong or a moral failing. Relying on alcohol to cope with stress or to socialize isn't inherently "good" or "bad." It's easy. In fact, it's just about the easiest thing you could do. And because of so much conditioning and repetition, drinking has become the ultimate comfort-zone behavior.

Had a bad day? Have a drink. Stressed from work? Open a bottle of wine. Celebrating a milestone? Let's go get drinks. Want to have fun? Drink. Relief from boredom? Drink. Feel relaxed and pampered? Drink. We outsource so much to alcohol, it's no wonder we feel incapable of tapping into those states on our own. It's a fast way to distract yourself, distance yourself from uncomfortable thoughts and emotions, and step into a false la-la land.

Drinking is hitting the big "ignore" button on the feelings and emotions you were meant to process, in order to grow and achieve the next stage of evolution in your development. Hanging out in your comfort zone isn't wrong. But when you let what's easy in the moment define your life's path, you're in for a lot of regret about what you could have done and who you could have become. Being able to process your feelings, to sit through this process and observe the feeling of being stressed after work, is how humans develop emotional resilience and become better able to cope with a wide spectrum of feelings, which in turn makes us more capable and successful in life. You might think you're muting what's hard, but you're really muting the opportunity to grow.

I want you to lean in. I want you to spend the next eight weeks with this framework in mind. At first, thinking your thoughts and feeling your emotions, instead of resorting to your typical coping mechanism, will feel awkward and uncomfortable. But you'll learn so much about yourself in the process and develop your capability. It won't always be easy. But screw easy. You're ready to challenge yourself outside of "easy" and find fulfilling instead. When you reflexively want to grab a drink for fill-in-the-blank reason, remember that you can learn to process your emotions in healthier ways, which makes you feel more connected, vibrant, and "enough."

And you're not alone. Your inner guide is with you. Your inner guide is who told you to pick up this book. Your inner guide believes you're capable of anything you set your mind to, and she will never lead you astray. Call it your intuition, your soul, your connection with source, God, the universe, or your higher self, your inner guide is a voice you can lean on for comfort, answers, and all-encompassing love and faith. She is the more inspired, more confident, more alive version of you. She doesn't see limitations. She recognizes danger, but she doesn't experience fear. She knows that you chose to be here on this planet to expand your consciousness, and she's here to guide you to your truest expression and purpose.

You can connect with your inner guide anytime. You connect with her through journaling, meditation and silence, moments of awe, being out in nature, and feel-good movement. Be on the lookout this week for signs that you're on the right path. Listening to your inner guide feels expansive, while listening to your fears feels restrictive. Fears usually manifest as excuses or "logical reasoning." Reflect on the times in your life you've been led by your inner guide versus your fear, and be present to what you think and feel now.

QUESTION YOUR
BELIEFS AROUND ALCOHOL

As I shared throughout the book, most of your beliefs around alcohol aren't serving you and who you want to become. Your beliefs, or reasons why you like to drink, are often passed down from society. They're a construct built by culture, billion-dollar marketing, and limiting beliefs about why you aren't enough on your own. I often meet with clients who share these constructs, which they picked up a long time ago—for example, the idea that nondrinkers are boring or not complex. It's an old-fashioned paradigm passed down since Prohibition in the 1920s, which keeps them stuck in a limiting pattern, for fear of seeming puritanical.

We all have cultural associations and normalized beliefs and behavior around drinking. As I've shown, drinking more than the health guidelines is the new normal. No one bats an eye at unlimited champagne brunch. Most regular drinkers don't just have one drink. Start looking around, and you'll see it too. This normalized behavior comes with strong messages about the role of alcohol in our lives:

- Every adult drinks.
- Drinking is normal.
- Drinking is a way to bond with others.
- Had a breakup or stressful day? Alcohol is there for you.
- Celebrating a milestone/going out with friends/ made it to the weekend? Drink.
- Only people whose lives are out of control quit drinking.
- Nondrinkers are boring.

It's up to you to decide if these beliefs are serving you. You can consciously choose to step out of the matrix and not believe any of this bullshit anymore. You could take your power back and believe things that empower you instead of disempower you. Believing that only people who hit rock bottom quit drinking was a belief that disempowered me for years. It forced me to stay stuck in a habit I know didn't make me happy, and for what reason? To keep my life small and keep up with appearances? To keep up with this unspoken expectation that normal adults drink? Drinking made me feel gross the next day and brought me a lot of stress and lost mornings. Yet I continued to justify its presence in my life because of the belief that drinking is normal. You know what else was normal a few decades ago? Smoking a pack of cigarettes. And today, so is feeling drained all the time or working a job that doesn't fulfill you. The people who defy the rules above are rebels.

My client Julie spent a lifetime telling herself limiting stories. She felt that her life's purpose revolved around raising children and bringing home a paycheck. It wasn't until she started getting clarity from exploring an alcohol-free life that she realized she was more than a "role" society had assigned to her. She had her own dreams. And she is finally awake to the fact that she doesn't need anyone's permission to go after them. Today, she's halfway through writing her first book, a dream she's had in her heart since she was a child. She works on herself every day and has expanded her gratitude, faith, courage, and passions. Her personal growth and development are just as important as anything else in her family.

In addition to normalized beliefs around alcohol, you also have reasons you like to drink—you think it brings you comfort, pleasure, or benefits. These are mental associations you've picked up and likely never questioned. This week's homework will help you gain a laser focus on the reasons you like drinking. Take the week to focus on the question "Why do I like to drink?," and try to list at least ten to fifteen reasons. Maybe you like to relax after a busy day, celebrate the weekend and let loose, make socializing easier, treat yourself, drink to fall asleep, or you like the taste.

As you go through the plan, you'll ask yourself, *Are these beliefs scientifically true? And do they empower or disempower me?* I've seen a great bumper sticker that speaks to this concept: "Don't believe everything you think." Life is a process of learning, unlearning, and relearning. And it's time to scrutinize your beliefs around drinking so that you can break the mental associations. Each of my reasons for drinking seemed innocuous and normal—it relaxes me, it's fun, it made socializing easier, and so on. But when I worded each belief differently, I knew they weren't 100 percent true:

- I can't relax without drinking.
- I'm no fun without alcohol.
- It's impossible for me to socialize without a drink.

Pretty disempowering, right? Each belief indicated that I didn't feel like I was enough on my own, without a chemical substance. I bet a version of these beliefs are anchored in your subconscious too. As we go on this eight-week break, you'll take your power back by disproving each limiting belief. For example, I may have thought that drinking made socializing easier because it gave me liquid courage. In reality, I was swimming in insecurities even while I was drinking. Alcohol didn't make me feel confident; it made me insecure and, toward the end of the night, disconnected.

Guess what I just did? I took a reason I thought I liked to drink and proved it's not fundamentally true. As I continue to reinforce my new belief (alcohol makes me insecure), my "reason" for drinking vanishes and slowly removes my desire. You believe what you reinforce, so are you ready to adopt new, empowering beliefs over the next eight weeks?

Keep your list of reasons handy. Because now, instead of merely pondering them, you get to experience a different way of being and see if any of them hold up. In week 4, with some new evidence in hand, you're going to revisit these beliefs and disprove each one.

DON'T GIVE IN TO FOMO

Life without alcohol isn't boring. It's fascinating to be fully present for life's full spectrum of experiences. But you need the proper mindset and tools to experience it this way, instead of feeling FOMO (fear of missing out). Think back on your life, before you started drinking. Did you experience fun back then? When you were young, you didn't need alcohol to enjoy birthday parties or school dances or sleepovers or ice skating. So why do you believe you need alcohol to have fun now?

Drinking might seem fun. It floods your brain with dopamine that your brain recognizes as enjoyable. It lets you be a passive zombie while fireworks go off up there. It's letting a beverage entertain you. But it's not engaging you in any way. Real fun is being an active participant and engaging fully in your life and experiences. Challenge yourself to think about how you can create fun in your life by engaging with the world around you. Instead of feeling FOMO, tap into JOMO—the joy of missing out. Feel joyful to miss out on hangovers and a depleted bank account, so you can fully experience life.

DEAL WITH CRAVINGS

As excited as you may be to change your life and transform your relationship with alcohol, I'm sure it won't be long before cravings rear their ugly head. All drinkers experience cravings in some form or another—it's what the repetitive action of drinking a beverage like alcohol does to your brain. Remember how alcohol affects the pleasure center and releases an artificially high level of dopamine. Over time, experience, and exposure, you've come to expect the reward of dopamine as tied to certain cues. Cue: You get home from work. Click: Your brain craves alcohol. Of course it does, because for years the cue has signaled that you're about to get a reward. When you experience a craving and don't give in, your brain doesn't get what it expected. And this can feel uncomfortable.

But nothing is wrong. Wanting is not an emergency situation. For years your brain has learned that it gets X reward with

Y situation, like a Pavlovian dog, but it can also unlearn this habit. Each time you crave alcohol, you can stop and try to understand the craving instead of giving in. In the moment, you may think alcohol will make you feel better. But does indulging truly make it better? How do you feel the next day? Has it led to long-term happiness? Does it allow you to process stress, or does it compound it?

Every craving you experience has an incredibly powerful piece of information for you, if you slow down and listen. It all starts with becoming more aware of your thoughts and feelings and becoming proactive instead of reactive. When you crave a drink, stop and assess what you're feeling and thinking. If you find yourself wanting a drink after a stressful day, analyze your feelings. Why was the day stressful? You do deserve to take a break and relax, but what other healthy ways could you relax and self-soothe that won't make you feel worse and even more stressed tomorrow? A nice tea, bath, and book?

Be curious and journal through the feelings and emotions that led to the craving. And keep in mind that a craving rarely lasts long, usually only twenty minutes.[2] Change your environment, and don't be scared to sit with the discomfort, because it means you're growing. It's like holding a yoga pose. Every time you learn to cope in a new way, you're laying down new neural pathways and weakening those associated with reaching for a drink.

PLAY OUT THE NIGHT

Imagine what it looks like to give in to your craving. Maybe you had an intense and stressful day at work with a ton of new follow-ups and to-dos for tomorrow. It's been go-go-go all day, and the first thing you do when you come home, without even thinking about it, is pour a glass of wine. One glass seems to sweep away your anxiety and stress, so you have another. And another.

Before you know it, the night is a total wash. You don't work out or eat well. You're barely present for homework and bedtime with your kids. You don't read that book you were planning to read. You end up on the couch watching Netflix. And you definitely don't write down the work follow-ups that are buzzing in your brain. The next day, you wake up with a pounding headache. You slept horribly and feel awful.

But worst of all is the shame. It's the umpteenth time you bailed on your diet and exercise plan. It's the umpteenth time you drank more than you wanted to. And staring down at you is the monumental scale of everything you have to do, but you have no stamina or courage to face it.

Yesterday you drank to deal with stress, but drinking compounded it and didn't address the source of the stress. In fact, drinking worsened your stress. Plus, all the little promises you broke to yourself add to the shame, regret, blame, and feelings of low self-esteem. It might not seem like a big deal, but this isn't the first time it's happened. It happens regularly enough for it to create some self-doubt. As though you can't entirely trust yourself to follow through with your own plans and needs.

IMAGINE A NEW OUTCOME

What if you revisit this exact scenario, but with a different outcome? Work is stressful. You come home and crave a drink, but instead, you take out your journal. Instead of masking your feelings, you work to uncover them by freewriting about the day, letting your unfiltered, unedited words fill the page—and you discover some insights. For instance, you love how much responsibility you're given at work, but you also feel taken advantage of when you work hard without additional pay or support. This process helps you learn things. Yes, you deserve to relax and unwind from stress, but you probably also need to improve your self-care and self-soothe to feel more appreciated and loved.

Imagine all the possible activities you could do to fill these two needs and to give yourself permission to relax. You could cook a delicious, healthy meal because you know you feel best when you nourish yourself. You could walk your dog and get out of your head and into nature. You could treat yourself with something that brings you joy, like a bubble bath or reading a new book. You could take all those work to-dos buzzing in your brain and write down next steps or plan a conversation with your boss. And you could even decompress with a drink—an alcohol-free one! Having addressed your source of stress, you can unplug and become engaged with your kids. When you go to bed that night, you feel at peace and well cared for, and easily fall asleep. The next morning, you wake up happy and respected because you didn't drink. You feel confident to tackle your day.

What a world of difference between those two scenarios. Yet how many times did I put myself through the first one? Over time, I'd taught my body and brain how to respond when I experienced stress: stress = wine. I repeated the cycle, and my brain learned. You must ingrain new patterns of behavior to handle your stress and examine your feelings. Here are some ideas.

INCORPORATE NEW RITUALS

Once you identify your cues, you can prepare a plan. If you find that you crave a drink on Fridays or after a stressful workday, have new rituals ready. Many of us are constantly on, striving to be productive and scrambling to accomplish our never-ending to-do lists. Drinking is often an excuse to finally turn off and a signal that it's time to relax.

But you can establish healthier ways to signal that the workday is done and set your mind to a new wavelength. You can create a ritual that says you deserve permission to relax, rest, and turn off, without numbing yourself and setting yourself up for worse feelings the next day. When you feel overwhelmed and need to let off steam from your go-go-go day, try these new rituals instead:

- Take a walk outside
- Watch the sunset
- Get your favorite take-out meal
- Sit in child's pose for a few minutes
- Do some yin yoga or qigong
- Listen to your favorite song and dance around your living room
- Call a friend, especially one who values growth and healthy habits
- Have a drink! You know, the kind without ethanol (get ideas below)

Try to incorporate at least one of these a few times this week, to mark the transition at the end of the day, and find what works for you.

I also want to tell you this: take it easy. The first two weeks without alcohol are no walk in the park. It takes your body time to detoxify, recalibrate, and rebalance to your natural rhythms. Some of my clients report headaches, fatigue, and even trouble sleeping. Give yourself extra grace and compassion during this time. Your body is healing on a massive level. Honor it. Take naps, sleep more than usual, don't push yourself to do a ton of things at one time, and let yourself feel proud of each day you accomplish.

MAKE IT FUN:
EXPLORE ALCOHOL-FREE DRINKS

In part I, I shared the explosive growth of new, alternative, alcohol-free drinks on the market. I want to remind you not to deprive yourself. If you use a drink to signal it's the weekend or to give yourself permission to relax, don't stop doing that. Treat yourself! Find an ethanol-free alternative that you love. A drink doesn't have to include a toxic substance for it to feel fun and special. Since I stopped drinking alcohol, I've become an amateur mocktail mixologist. I love to experiment with different flavors and natural ingredients. My clients also love experimenting with alcohol-free drinks. It feels like having your cake and eating it too. Enjoying new nonalcoholic drinks doesn't force you to completely overhaul your habit of treating yourself with a beverage. Don't stop treating yourself—just change the treat.

Here are some ideas:

- Make a new favorite at home. Try a new mocktail recipe from this book or my blog, try drinks like Spindrift or San Pellegrino Sparkling Juices, or mix your favorite juice with sparkling water.
- At a restaurant or bar, order club soda with bitters, ginger beer with lime, or ask the waiter for the restaurant's best mocktails. Restaurants and cocktail bars have been stepping it up in the last few years.

Find restaurants that already have mocktails or other nonalcoholic drinks you like on their menus.

- Explore nonalcoholic craft brews or prepared mocktails. By the time this book goes to press, there will no doubt be dozens of drinks on the market. Some fan favorites today include Curious Elixirs, Kin Euphorics, Saint Ivy, Surreal Brewing, Athletic Brewing, and Gruvi. Miss your favorite wine? Try Ariel or Botanique.

WEEK 1 MOCKTAIL

SPICY GINGER MANGO

I had a version of this mocktail at a hip restaurant in Vancouver and re-created the flavors at home. Spicy and tropical—I love it!

MAKES 1 SERVING

- 120ml ginger beer
- 90ml mango juice
- Juice of half a lemon
- 3–4 slices fresh jalapeño

- Ice
- Sparkling water, to taste
- Dash of ginger bitters, if desired

Put the ginger beer, mango juice, lemon juice, and 2–3 jalapeño slices in a cocktail shaker with ice and shake vigorously. Pour the mixture over ice in a glass and add sparkling water to your liking. Top with ginger bitters, if desired. Garnish with one jalapeño slice.

USE TRACKING TO GIVE
YOURSELF A HIT OF DOPAMINE

Scientists have discovered that making progress on your goals releases dopamine, even for small goals and achievements.[3] Ever heard of quick wins? Quick wins are small goals that you can easily accomplish that give you the momentum and belief to keep going and accomplish bigger goals. Our brains release dopamine when we check any item on our list as done. No wonder I've always loved checklists and bullet journals (I have four to six journals at a time to keep track of my goals and interests). Dopamine is both a pleasure and motivation neurotransmitter that will help you repeat actions that elicit its release in the first place. So, instead of using it to your disadvantage with alcohol, use it to your advantage with tracking. For example, have you ever started an exercise plan and stuck with it for a while, so you could log it later in an app or journal? That's the effect of this kind of motivation. I'm a big fan of tracking.

You know how sometimes you wake up in the morning with the best intentions, and things get harder later in the evening? Use that to your advantage. Take out a calendar and, in the morning, make a checkmark for not drinking that day, before you're tempted later in the evening. In fact, put a calendar in a few different places—your desk, fridge, or on your person— and, in the morning, mark off in three different places that you didn't drink that day. By the time the evening comes around, along with its temptations, you'll be less likely to drink because you won't want to have to go back and cross off your progress in all these places. To this day, I use this method for many of my goals. For example, when I commit to meatless eating for a time, I don't wait to decide what I'll do when someone offers me a slice of pepperoni pizza (I love pizza). In the morning I'd already checked off that I didn't eat meat, so that pepperoni pizza no longer registers as an option. Check out www.euphoricaf.com/book-bonus to get a free calendar for your tracking.

YOUR JOURNALING HOMEWORK

Excellent job this week! You're amazing! Before the week's end, answer the following questions in your journal:

1. Why do you *like* to drink? List all the reasons you like to drink alcohol—for example, *I like to relax and unwind after a busy week, I like to treat myself, I like to socialize with alcohol,* and so on. Try to tease out all the reasons you believe you enjoy drinking and keep this list handy for week 4. By then, you'll have enough evidence to prove that these reasons may not be entirely true.

2. What cues lead you to want to drink? Stress? The weekend? 5:00 p.m.? Vacation? Socializing? List all of your cues. What new rituals will you incorporate instead? List as many as you can think of.

3. What does it feel like to give in to a craving? How do you feel a few hours later or the next day? Did acting on the craving make you feel more fulfilled? The next time you have a craving, take out a journal and describe it and what events or feelings led to it.

4. List at least five things you're grateful for this week.

Let Go of Shame

RECOGNIZE THAT IT'S NOT YOUR FAULT

You wake up groggy with a slight headache and stale, dry breath. It's Monday morning, and last night you drank too much wine while watching TV, trying to delay the Sunday blues. You feel like you've been run over by a truck. But what really upsets you is how freaking disappointed you are for being in this state again. You vow you can't keep waking up like this. You can't keep putting your life on hold to deal with these hangovers and low moods. You vow that you won't drink again for a while, or at least not tonight. Somehow you make it through the day, with no energy or love for anyone, and crash as soon as you can. You lay off the wine for a few days, and the week improves. You start your workout routine again, you cook healthy meals, and you start to feel great!

Then, it's Thursday night, and you've been invited out for sushi with friends. Sushi always calls for sake and beer. This isn't you sitting at home drinking wine alone and watching TV. Come on—you've been good all week, and you deserve it. But only two drinks. You go out, but two drinks turns into three—everyone is having a third—plus another beer when you get home, as a nightcap. You had a fun night with your friends! But five short hours later, you wake up at 4:00 a.m., and the night hits you like a truck again.

The above scenario may have played out differently for you. Maybe you had this battle every day, every few days, or every weekend. What matters here is the duality of desires. Part of you (the part that picked up this book) has wanted to take a break or go alcohol-free. This is your conscious, intuitive mind. It's driven by your higher self and looks out for your future contentment. It creates goals and drives you to work on self-improvement. This is your human brain, or neocortex. It evolved seventy thousand years ago and made humans the thinkers, planners, and doers that we are today.

But your subconscious, instinctual mind? That's still there too. We all have mid- and lower-brains that evolved from reptilian times. This part of your brain is driven by survival and mental associations that are strengthened with repetition. And because alcohol, with its release of dopamine, tricks your brain into thinking alcohol is important for survival, you have two competing desires. You've wanted to drink less or not at all for a while, yet your subconscious mind still yearns to drink.

Many forces are at play in a routine drinking habit—habit formation, alcohol's addictive quality, societal conditioning, personal relevance, and neuro-associative beliefs. However, because we don't understand these forces, it's easy to fall into intense shame and blame for desires and actions around drinking. This week we'll focus on learning more about these invisible forces, so you can let go of the shame and completely forgive yourself.

HABIT LOOPS

Most of our habits are outside our conscious awareness. That's why they're habits. We don't have to think about or remind ourselves to do them. They happen almost reflexively. How does an action or activity become a habit? And how can we change our habits?

I want you to think back on your life and guess how many times you've drank. I don't ask you to do this to make you feel bad; my own number must be in the thousands. I ask you to do it to show you the power of repetitive actions on your brain. You didn't drink a few times here and there over your lifetime. It's something you've done on autopilot for years, decades even! And each time you drank, you laid down a tiny, thin thread in your brain. Drink here, drink there, and more thin threads are laid down, until the thread thickens. Drink a thousand times, and the thread turns to rope. This desire is firmly rooted throughout various neural pathways and, when you repeat the action, it automatically gets absorbed into your subconscious and rooted as a habit in your basal ganglia.

Neuroscientist Marc Lewis shows that this is essentially what happens with alcohol use and our neural pathways, in his book *The Biology of Desire: Why Addiction Is Not a Disease*. Our brains aren't wrong—they're doing exactly what they were meant to do with a drink like alcohol: form strong habits and neural pathways around it! But you are not your habits. You are not your unhealthy patterns. Every habit that isn't serving you and who you want to become can be unlearned. The rope can be unraveled, and it helps to understand how habit loops are formed, so you can change them.

Charles Duhigg, author of *The Power of Habit: Why We Do What We Do in Life and Business*, explains that habits are made up of three components: the cue, the activity, and the reward. The *cue* is your trigger, and it tells your brain to go into autopilot mode. A cue for drinking could be coming home from work, dining out, Friday night, passing the wine aisle, feeling stressed, 5:00 p.m., and so on. The *activity* is what you engage in—pouring a drink and drinking it. And the *reward* is the benefit you associate with the activity, the momentary release of dopamine or putting your worries to the wayside. Over time, Duhigg explains, "The cue and reward become intertwined until a powerful sense of anticipation and craving emerges."[1] The cues signal that it's time for megareward, and your brain stops making decisions at that point.

While disrupting your habits isn't easy, understanding this cycle can help you "hack" the system. Plenty of people strong-arm their way into a break from alcohol and only focus on not having a drink—an ultimate game of willpower. They constantly experience cues and have to white-knuckle through them. Nevertheless, cues never go away because your triggers are normal parts of your day and week. It will eventually be 5:00 p.m. on a Friday; you can't escape that. The key in changing your habit is replacing the activity with something that will give you a similar reward. That's why I'm a big proponent of alcohol-free drinks. It's an easy switch. You can still reward yourself or decompress over a drink, just one that doesn't have ethanol in it. You can also experiment with all kinds of activities that make you feel good. Soon enough, new patterns will override your old habits.

Habit change, especially breaking a bad habit, takes disruption, momentum, and commitment. It's almost like a rocket launch. It takes a lot of effort to get the rocket launched through the Earth's atmosphere, but once it hits space, its movement becomes effortless. There's a point where freedom and new habit patterns carry you. That's why I always recommend taking a break from drinking for a set number of days (commit, disrupt, and gain momentum) and why you're doing an eight-week challenge. The time period is more than long enough to disrupt your habits and give you the opportunity to replace old patterns with new ones.

NEURO-ASSOCIATIVE BELIEFS

Uncovering and deconstructing your beliefs around drinking is a major purpose of this book. Your reasons for drinking and why you believe it gives you pleasure, comfort, or benefits are at the crux of the desire. These beliefs are also buried within your subconscious, because the subconscious makes these life-long neuro-associations, such as *Drinking helps me relax* or *I have to drink while watching the game.* When I still drank, I consciously knew that I felt horrible after drinking, yet somehow, it kept happening to me. My desire to change was strong on Monday morning but completely unsustainable and disappeared by the weekend. I believed that something must be terribly wrong with me and my self-control and willpower. I spiraled into negative ruminations and felt at odds with myself. Half the time I hated myself for drinking more than I wanted to; the other half I told myself how much I deserved to be treated.

The cognitive dissonance that you're learning about is pure mental anguish. It's like a never-ending war filled with suffering and futility. But you can get out from under your competing desires—you're working on that right now. By introducing new concepts and frameworks to understand your drinking habit, you're breaking free of the two dominant thought patterns you have around it: *I love drinking/I hate drinking. I want to drink less/I want a glass of wine after work.* You're also learning to dissociate alcohol with pleasure. All animals gravitate toward pleasure and away from pain. That's what your lower- and mid-brains are meant to do. During your life, you've associated pleasure with drinking and pain with not being able to drink. I did too.

But today I link pleasure to fulfillment, happiness, well-being, and growth (all things incongruent with drinking). I link pleasure to deep restorative sleep, living authentically as the real me, going after my dreams, and being an alcohol-free rebel in a world that tells us we have to drink. I link pain to acting inauthentically under the effect of alcohol. I link pain to hangovers. I link pain to having a beverage control me. I link pain to the disempowering beliefs that say I need alcohol. As you continue with this journey, you'll attach new associations with drinking and new associations with alcohol-free living. You are slowly changing what you link pain and pleasure to and tricking your reptilian brain into aligning with your higher consciousness.

ALCOHOL'S ADDICTIVE NATURE

Alcohol isn't just psychologically addictive—it's also chemically addictive. According to the National Institute of Drug Abuse, alcohol is considered one of the five most addictive drugs to the human brain, more addictive than nicotine and methamphetamines.[2] Only heroin and cocaine rank as more addictive than alcohol, something we drink all the time and don't think twice about.

As you've learned, alcohol immediately affects the pleasure center in your brain and releases an artificially high level of dopamine, something we evolutionarily chase. It's how we survive (think food and sex). Over time, your exposure to drinking also changes the way you feel when the alcohol effects wear off. Have you ever had a few drinks, stopped drinking, and didn't go to bed right away? Maybe you had a few at brunch or a celebratory lunch and then had to continue on with your day. How did you feel two hours after drinking? I bet pretty low, groggy, and tired.

Remember that while alcohol releases dopamine and depresses our central nervous system, your body releases stress hormones like cortisol to counteract that effect. When it's hard to stop after one drink, not only does your body crave the next hit of dopamine, it also wants to evade the crash that follows. This is a normal response to alcohol. Look around you. Most regular drinkers have more than one drink. Your brain wants more pleasure and less pain in the moment, and the anesthetic effect of alcohol numbs the parts of your brain that control judgment and self-control. Good intentions don't stand a chance here.

So instead of separating "problem" drinkers from "normal" ones, what if we started to recognize that alcohol is addictive to humans? What if we started to rightly assign blame to the drink and not the drinker? What if we stopped letting the alcohol industry get away with the narrative that you're the problem, and that the product isn't the problem? Think of the way we consider cigarette smokers. Most people understand that once you start smoking, especially at a young age, you can get addicted and it's hard to quit. We don't blame smokers; it's the way nicotine works on the body. If you become dependent on alcohol, which most routine drinkers are to some extent, society makes it seem like something is wrong with you, like you have some kind of genetic mutation, as if alcohol isn't an addictive substance. I work with women who drink no more than one or two glasses of wine at a time, yet when they come to me, they're mentally locked on the habit. It has a strong pull, regardless of the quantity. We must start talking about alcohol in a different way.

SOCIETAL CONDITIONING AND MARKETING

When I was getting my MBA, I had a society and law professor who shared a brilliant observation. Businesses are always looking to get new users and expand their consumer base: customer acquisition. Yet when you look at, say, the cigarette industry, it looks like an uphill battle. The likelihood of persuading a forty-year-old nonsmoker with peer pressure, marketing, and messaging to start smoke cigarettes is slim. My professor joked that it would be a ridiculous proposal for anyone to convince him to start smoking at this point in his life. So what does the industry do? They target young people. They create a perception of smoking as cool, rebellious, and a sign of independence. Teenagers are their target market for new customers. Not so coincidently, when do most of us start drinking?

Whether it's to fit in, prove independence, or feel like an adult, drinking is a rite of passage in our younger years. Many women I work with started drinking in college and developed strong habits then, and while they may have tamed their habits as they moved into adulthood, they never really changed them. It's ridiculous to think that our eighteen-year-old selves dictate our life habits. What an outdated relationship! Even if you don't start in high school or college, in our society, the likelihood of becoming a drinker is high. Imagine what a person would have to do to evade it. They'd have to evade drinking as teenagers experimenting; in college at college parties; at new jobs going out with coworkers for happy hour; on the dating scene; with career advancement and having wine dinners with clients and executives; in motherhood, when mommy circles peddle "mommy juice"; or in retirement, while trying to fill the time. You'd have to evade it at dinner parties, networking events, cookouts, fancy restaurants, nights out with your friends, holidays, and the list goes on. Unless you live somewhere alcohol consumption is prohibited, at some point you're in an environment where drinking regularly is the norm.

And then there's big alcohol, a $252 billion-per-year industry.[3] It promises you good vibes and laughter on the Corona commercial; it shows you as a refined and sophisticated foodie on a food and wine show. It's rosé-all-day tinted Instagram accounts, it's craft breweries on every street corner, and it's even sponsoring wellness events and marathon races. While marketing regulations have gotten stricter about what alcohol companies can say, the advertisements still easily imply that drinking makes you more sociable and popular. During the COVID-19 pandemic, many ads promoted drinking to handle stress, a dangerous message.

The alcohol industry spends billions of dollars marketing alcohol and research has shown that it employs similar tactics to those the tobacco industry once used. A recent report in *The Counter* also showed that the industry spreads misinformation about alcohol's health risks. The report found a long history of the industry's efforts to obstruct the truth about alcohol's health risks, including funding research that makes it look healthy. As Nigel Brockton, vice president of research at the American Institute for Cancer Research, says: "The tobacco industry pioneered this by manipulating the science on heart disease and cancer, by hiring researchers who pretty much get on their payroll and then create doubt about the linkages."[4] The alcohol industry relies on the myth that moderate drinking is heart healthy—a myth perpetuated by flawed studies that drew limited conclusions that have now been thoroughly debunked. Creating doubt and ambiguity is the point. It's to keep you unaware.

In the past two decades, marketing alcohol to women has gotten a lot more aggressive. There are low-calorie cocktails and sayings like "wine o'clock," and this pervasive idea that wine is self-care, or worse, mommy juice. When shopping, maybe you've seen products with sayings like "Here's to wine, because yoga can only do so much" or "The most expensive part of having kids is all the wine you have to drink." These might seem funny or cute, but they aren't. Women need connection, well-being, growth, support, and a society that values their work and contribution. They don't need alcohol to handle life—they deserve much better. Alcohol advertising preys on the fact that women are overstressed and do more labor with less compensation, by offering a negative solution that makes it harder to cope over time.

Now that you understand how all these sneaky forces are at play, breathe a huge sigh of relief. Most of us don't know how alcohol works on our brains and how powerful conditioning is. Instead, we're made to feel that something is wrong with us and that we're broken. So get ready to let go of shame, own your story, and forgive yourself for the past.

SAY YOUR TRUTH
AND ACCEPT YOUR STORY

Shame lingers not only in the embarrassing nights and inauthentic conversations. It also lies in disowning parts of yourself. Being able to realize that you're not alone and that you don't need to keep hiding this part of yourself removes a huge burden. Shame cannot survive when it's spoken about—it cannot survive telling the truth and being honest with ourselves. Shame grows in secret and festers in our minds. Our vulnerability is the antidote to shame.

In my first month of living alcohol-free, I flocked to private Facebook groups to talk out my new discoveries and express my feelings. I found thousands of people who felt the same. In these groups, people shared their stories and their epiphanies and insights on changing their relationship with alcohol. They shared moments of pride, gratitude, and self-esteem. This is owning the entire human experience. When I kept everything secret, I was allowing parts of me to grow into a complete lack of faith in myself, my capabilities, and my worthiness as a human being. Keeping it hidden made me believe I was a screwup instead of an imperfect, authentic human seeking love and connection. As cliché as it may sound, the truth really will set you free. I'd love to invite you to join the private Euphoric Facebook group, to share your perspective and relate to others: www.euphoricaf.com/book-bonus.

You need to know that you were doing the best you could with the tools and information you had at the time. You didn't fail at self-control or willpower or have some kind of character flaw. It's time to completely forgive yourself. Memories that hold shame and guilt are a weight on your shoulders and taking up precious mental space. Everything unpleasant and painful that's happened to you serves at least one purpose: to show you exactly what you don't want more of in your life. This can seem obvious, but think about it. Most people don't know what they want in their lives—and you have these experiences that point to exactly what you don't want more of. You get to choose again. In fact, you have the rest of your life to choose again. Start by fully accepting yourself and your experiences (thank you for the lessons!) and owning your truth. Again, it's realizing that all of it served a purpose and that your experiences are not shameful, sinful, amoral, or even unique. When you own your story, it stops having power over you.

Even the act of journaling—which I know you're doing a great job with!—can help you own your story and accept yourself. My client Emma found a lot of relief by putting pen to paper. Journaling helps acknowledge and affirm your story, and while it might feel private, maybe one day you'll share your journey with your partner or best friend. Who knows? Maybe one day you'll share your story outspokenly and openly. When you work on embracing your story, one day you won't feel shame. Breaking free from the silence is liberating.

WEEK 2 MOCKTAIL

PINEAPPLE TIKI DRINK

Spiced tea is a revelation. It adds so much body to a drink and can be used to replace rum in any tiki-style cocktail. Treat yourself with a comforting and indulgent mocktail made with spiced tea:

MAKES 1 SERVING

- 90ml spiced tea, like chai or Bengal, steeped and cooled
- 120ml pineapple juice
- 45ml cream of coconut
- 30ml orange juice
- Ice

Put the spiced tea, pineapple juice, cream of coconut, and orange juice in a shaker with ice and shake vigorously. Pour the mixture over ice in a tall glass and garnish with a tiki umbrella or a flower.

YOUR JOURNALING HOMEWORK

Forgiveness is meant for you every time you've let yourself down or for anything you've done that you regret. It's an important step to embrace yourself for who you've been, love yourself for who you are, and forgive yourself for your shortcomings. You were doing the best you could, and all of it brought you here today.

There's an old Hawaiian prayer, called the Ho'oponopono prayer, that you can recite to clear the negative energy, process and heal what needs to be processed and healed, and release your shame to the universe, so it leaves you with less emotional charge.

Find a quiet place and sit down with your journal. Play some relaxing music and light a candle. Take a moment and inhale deeply for the count of four. Hold for the count of four. Release on the count of four. Repeat four more times. Let yourself relax. *Breathe.* Think of the memory or aspect of yourself that brings you pain and shame. Say the prayer aloud to yourself: "I forgive you. I'm sorry. Thank you. I love you."

Now grab your journal, write down each phrase, and expand upon each one with a few sentences.

- I forgive (the shame-inducing experience—write it all down)
- I'm sorry (for my contribution to it)

- Thank you (for what it taught me or where I am now because of it)
- I love you (for doing the best I could with the tools I had/ for being a wholly imperfect human, etc.)

Last, write your name and the words: "I forgive myself. I was doing the best I could with the information I had. I am learning and growing in ways that are new, and I forgive the past version of myself who didn't have these tools." When you finish, repeat the prayer again—"I forgive you. I'm sorry. Thank you. I love you"—as you think of this memory and release it.

Lots of emotional work this week! Your bravery inspires me. While this week's topics were challenging, I hope the introspection gives you an emotional release. You owe yourself forgiveness and freedom from shame or blame.

Step into Your Best Health

YOUR BODY IS HEALING

Your body's been going through a lot of changes, and you're on a massive healing journey. Don't forget what you've learned about how fast the body can heal. Within a matter of weeks, studies on abstinence show that gray matter regrows in the brain, neurons regenerate, liver fat heals, cancer markers decrease, and blood pressure and cholesterol go down. Your body truly is a miracle. It's dealt with all the toxins thrown at it, and now you're treating it with so much love. Taking a break from alcohol might be one of the healthiest things you could do.

Don't feel that great yet? Stick with it. Because your body is recalibrating and healing, you may not have felt your best physically these first two weeks. But you're on your way out of this phase and into feeling exponentially better as each week passes. Let's use this week to reflect on your health journey, your habits, and nourishing yourself in a loving way. This one change can be the beginning of a domino effect to take care of yourself and your body. This eight-week plan isn't about changing a zillion things at once—it's not about taking a break from alcohol *and* going vegan *and* waking up at 5.00 a.m. every day to run four miles. It's about making gentle and intuitive shifts to your health, leading to healing and happiness.

REBALANCING YOUR SLEEP

After working with hundreds of people through a guided break from alcohol, I've learned that your sleep cycles are one of the most unique things about you. Each alcohol-free day and week allows your body to recalibrate and find its natural rhythms. I hope you find that your sleep is improving daily, but don't fret if it's not. While some do experience delicious, nourishing sleep within the first two weeks, many others find it takes many weeks longer. Everyone is different and has different drinking habits that their body is normalizing from. My client Simon was concerned that he wasn't sleeping well in the first few weeks but then turned a corner. By his fourth week alcohol-free, his sleep improved so much and he felt way more energetic. Now he feels so good he even takes a cold shower in the morning.

William Porter, author of *Alcohol Explained*, gave a great analogy in the *Euphoric* podcast episode we did together: Imagine you work an early shift and have to wake up at 4:00 a.m. every day for years. Then, you change jobs and can wake up at a more normal hour. Guess what? Your body is still conditioned to wake up at 4:00 a.m., even without using an alarm clock. Because alcohol induces the body to release stress hormones, and we feel these effects most in the wee hours of the night, your body has gotten used to being awakened and having fragmented sleep around this time. Even when the stress hormones aren't there, the pattern in your sleep cycles is. Have grace, love, and compassion for yourself and your body right now. If you can, sleep more than you're used to.

If you find it hard to fall asleep, here are some holistic tips that have worked for my clients:

- Avoid caffeine after 1:00 p.m., including caffeinated tea. (My tea cabinet is entirely full of noncaffeinated blends, since I drink tea at night.)
- Limit the amount of food you eat three hours before bed, or make a hard-and-fast rule that you stop eating at 7:00 p.m.
- Make going to bed a ritual. Put down any work or entertainment and do two to three routine activities that signal to your body that it's time to go to bed. For example, you could take a lavender bubble bath, drink a bedtime tea or golden milk (milk with turmeric and ginger from India—I drink mine plant-based), or listen to some meditation music or a sleep story.
- Cut yourself off from your phone or any other screens one to two hours before bed. Bring an old-fashioned book into the bedroom instead. Challenge yourself to read a hundred pages.
- Wear a sleep mask.
- Try to go to bed at the same time every night and wake up at the same time every morning. If you're having trouble falling asleep, try waking up earlier than usual.
- Wear socks to bed. Warm feet help you fall asleep. I can never fall asleep with cold feet.

If you wake up in the middle of the night and can't fall back asleep, try not to get frustrated. Instead, use the extra time to meditate or do a breathing technique: Breathe in through your mouth on the count of four, hold for a count of seven, release, and completely exhale through your mouth to the count of eight. Repeat the cycle at least four times.

Be patient. Alcohol has been messing with your circadian rhythm for decades. It will rebalance. Today, I go to bed early and wake up early, and I love it. I fall asleep within minutes and sleep deeply through the entire night. Every night, I get excited about falling asleep. I drift off while visualizing my goals and telling myself to remember my dreams, then wake up in the morning exploring them. It's fun.

GET NOURISHED

When you wake up feeling well rested and energized, food starts to take on a new quality. I know that part of you was motivated to read this book because you want to feel healthier and live longer. You can make some incredible holistic lifestyle changes as you shift your relationship with alcohol. But remember: this isn't a diet plan or fitness challenge, and I encourage you to be gentle with how many changes you're making at once. I'd love to share easy strategies that have worked for me and my clients to feel even better and create an upward spiral of well-being and health. Often, the biggest constraint to eating well is time, so here are the ways I fit healthy eating into my busy lifestyle. I suggest trying one new thing. Or just focus on your alcohol-free journey as it feels right for you. Your intuition gets to decide.

- Add more food groups rather than taking any away. Try not to make anything else off limits right now. When you make everything in your life all or nothing at once, it's not sustainable. Instead of worrying about avoiding foods that aren't the best for me, like cookies or doughnuts, I have a strategy of adding more healthy foods to my diet. Foods to add are any type of fruit and vegetable, especially water-rich fruits and vegetables. I use the app Daily Dozen to focus on the foods I can add into my day. This app provides a list of foods that the American Society for Nutrition (nutrition.org), the largest independent research body on nutrition, has devised to help people eat in the healthiest way possible. The daily dozen includes legumes, fruits, vegetables, whole grains, seeds, nuts, and spices, and you check off boxes throughout the day. It's like a game.

- Try to eat the same thing every day before 5:00 p.m., which makes it easier to choose healthy staples and ensure your nutritional needs are met. When you focus on adding instead of eating less in general (as most diet plans advise), your appetite gets satiated, and your body loves you. Here's a sample day of eating in my life:

> I intermittent fast and eat my breakfast for lunch. At that time, I'll make a bowl of oats, blueberries, banana, plant-based milk, and a blend of superfoods: flax (for omega 3s), turmeric (cancer fighting), and cinnamon (to reduce heart disease risk). I also make a green smoothie and have included the recipe for you at the end of this week 3 section.

> For a snack, I'll eat a tangerine, apple slices, some nuts, or tortilla chips with hummus.

Before I sit down for dinner, I snack on baby tomatoes and baby carrots. By dinner time, I've already eaten five or six servings of fruits and vegetables.

For dinner, I include a salad or cruciferous veggie. And for dessert, I might eat more fruit. This doesn't mean I don't eat pizza or enchiladas or cookies. I just try to ensure my necessities are met, so I don't feel guilty about having more indulgent items. Add more healthy items and worry less.

- Above all else, listen to your body. Eat intuitively and listen to what your body wants. When they begin the program, many of my clients struggle with snacking more often. Do you think you're snacking more too? It's normal. You might not be eating enough food at your mealtimes. Think of it this way: When you were drinking, your body was used to processing anywhere from 400 to 2,000-plus extra calories a week. If you weren't actively gaining weight, you were probably eating less to begin with, to accommodate those extra calories. Your meal portions might actually be way too small. Eat more at mealtimes, especially the good stuff.
- Drink teas and water with lemon. Hibiscus tea is great for lowering blood pressure, and green tea is good for improving your liver health. Lemon water is great to flush out your system. You can also drink green juices.

— SUGAR CRAVINGS —

Do you feel like you've turned into the Cookie Monster lately? If so, hurray! You've arrived. Sugar cravings are a rite of passage when you take a break from alcohol. After all, alcohol is produced from fermented sugar. Most alcohols are made from fruits or otherwise high glycemic foods (grapes, sugar cane, agave, barley). In addition, aside from the alcohol content, most drinks still have tons of extra sugar. Like alcohol, sugar releases a high spike of dopamine. So it's more than normal to crave sugar when you go alcohol-free. And I don't want you to go crazy trying to push that urge down.

When I gave up drinking, I remember one week that sugar cravings drove me nuts. I was reaching for sugar every night and was worried it was a new bad habit I'd have forever. One night, I told myself no sugar, and it was an intense night. But you know what? The sugar cravings lessen over time. You won't be a Cookie Monster for the rest of your life. My clients love gummy bears, so go grab some! Even so, here are some sweet snack ideas that might feel healthier:

- Try some dried fruit. I love dried mango. Many health food stores sell fruit bars that taste just like a fruit snack.
- Stock up on some vitamin gummies. With a multivitamin, vitamin D, and vitamin B gummy collection, you'll have several gummies a day with low sugar content.
- Make brownies or cake and replace the butter or oil with applesauce.
- Bake your own desserts from scratch. You can always make healthy swaps or lower the sugar content. And the

> fact that you're baking means it's not super convenient or mindless—it's a labor of love that gives you a little infusion of joy.

MOVE YOUR BODY AND BREATHE

In week 3, many of my clients start to feel things they've never felt before, such as emotions they didn't realize were there. Alcohol is an anesthetic. For as long as you've been drinking, it's been numbing your feelings, thoughts, and emotions. This means that when you take away the numbing agent, you're left with pure emotions. Ones that you might not be used to processing or feeling. Depending on your situation, this can feel amazing. You might feel profound moments of joy, gratitude, appreciation, and love. But it can also feel raw, like you've been unmasked, and your nerve endings are feeling unfamiliar sensations. Negative emotions, like anger, sadness, or fear, might surface as well.

In week 5, we'll do a deep dive into the story behind your emotions and what they're trying to tell you. But this week, I want to offer you three tools that are always at your disposal for dealing with raw emotions.

- *Journal.* Grab your journal and dissect what you're feeling. What emotion is it? What happened before you noticed it? Now that you recognize it, what do you need to process? Writing through emotions like this gives you the power of awareness and clarity, which then brings resolution. Let yourself do a freewrite to fully express yourself.

- *Breathe.* We are notoriously shallow breathers and don't recognize how important breath can be in changing our mental state. After all, oxygen is the number one element we need to survive. I highly recommend the Wim Hof method and his free app. The box method of breathing is really easy too. Just breathe in for the count of four, hold for the count of four, exhale for the count of four, and hold for the count of four. Repeat at least ten times.
- *Move.* Emotions are stored in our bodies and need to be processed with our bodies. Because emotions are bodily reactions triggered by neurotransmitters and hormones, changing the state of your body has the ability to change the state of your mind.

Moving your body doesn't mean you have to go through an intense sixty-day boot-camp regimen. Allow yourself to discover what feels good for you and what your body is craving. I started with yoga and a lot of hiking. I loved walking my dog in the hills by my house with a newfound appreciation. I also highly recommend dancing it out. Dance is primal. Our ancestors have been doing it for thousands of years. Dancing is a great way to shake it off, whether it's stress or a negative emotion, and also gives you a huge boost of happiness and enthusiasm. I often dance to an upbeat song as I'm waiting for my coffee to brew in the morning. I also dance when I'm celebrating a win, big or small. Bonus points: you can do it anytime and don't have to put on a sports bra. Whether it's through dance, walks, or yoga, moving your body is important for your mental health to release tension, anxious thoughts, and get those feel-good endorphins.

Though I started with a lot of gentle hikes, within six months I craved more endurance and stamina. I always envied people who were aerobically fit—long-distance runners amaze me. Yet I assumed I hated running. I could run a mile or two or do a 5K every few years, but never did I imagine myself running for hours. It looked way too uncomfortable, and I was happy to leave that feat to the runners in my life—my sister, husband, best friend, and cousins all ran full and half-marathons.

During my first year alcohol-free, I discovered I was far more capable than the stories I'd made up about myself. So, I decided to go for it—train and run a half-marathon. On my first few runs, when I desperately wanted to stop, I reminded myself that this was a lot like ditching alcohol: it was uncomfortable at first, but those moments of discomfort translated to much longer lasting pride and joy afterward.

I spent that half-year training and jogging around lakes and going on run dates with my husband. Before I knew it, I ran 13.1 miles and cried when I crossed the finish line. Along with having fun Friday nights without alcohol, running that distance wasn't something I thought I was capable of. Challenging yourself feels good. My clients pick up new, active hobbies like spinning, aerial yoga, kitesurfing, and CrossFit. It's exciting to explore what your body is capable of when drinking doesn't hold it back. Have fun and stop "shoulding" yourself about exercise. You're allowed to listen to your body and be gentle instead of trying to "fix" yourself. Below are some of my favorite ideas for moving your body:

- Go on a nice, long walk around your neighborhood.
- Explore local hikes in your area.
- Put on your favorite song and dance like a wild woman.
- Try a high-intensity interval workout or a new class.
- Relax with a yin yoga routine.

FEELING BORED

As you settle into a new norm and a new way of taking care of yourself, you might find you have a lot more time on your hands. *What if I get bored?* I get this question in some form or another from my clients and community a lot. And it's completely valid, because drinking takes up a lot of time. Maybe the act of drinking itself accounted for only 10 to 15 percent of your time, but there's much more to account for: the time it takes for alcohol to wear off, the time you're planning happy hour, the time you spend going to the store, the time you criticize yourself for drinking more than you want to, the time you make new rules to stick to, the time you worry about it, and the time you're feeling sick, low, and exhausted after drinking. Taking a break from alcohol frees up a lot of time and mental space! It's up to you to be creative about how to use your reclaimed time.

It's typical to feel restless with all this newfound time, especially at first. If you're used to drinking sometime between 5:00 and 10:00 p.m., you'll rack your brain, stumped with what you're supposed to do now. Think back to being a kid and what you did when you were bored. You probably climbed trees and put on plays and made up fantasies to your heart's content. But as adults, we've taught ourselves to reach for external stimulation, like TV, social media, and drinking. Drinking is one of the most passive things you can do—it's letting a beverage entertain you and release fireworks in your brain. Hence, why you feel so bored without it. But this is a great thing! It means that your brain is craving more internal stimuli, such as using your imagination and challenging yourself to do something interesting and perplexing. It means you have big ideas up there that are waiting to be expressed.

Boredom is the starting point of creativity. It might feel uncomfortable, but if you never felt bored, you also would never feel driven to create or build something new.

When you feel bored, the last thing you need is to watch TV or scroll through social media. You were meant to engage and actively participate in your own entertainment. Challenge yourself to do something you find enticing but have no idea how to do. For instance, my client Caroline picked up boxing. Like real-life, fight-for-your-life-in-a-hardcore-gym boxing. I'm amazed at the ways she's trying new things and becoming a student of new activities. Who knows where your new activity could take you? It could be as complicated as coding or as simple as drawing. You might discover a new world of passions and find a project that motivates, excites, scares, or challenges you. Check out www.euphoricaf.com/book-bonus for more ideas about how to spend your time.

WHAT IF I SLIP?

While the goal is to take an eight-week break from alcohol, your progress (and not perfection) is all that matters. If you slip and drink, keep going. Changing your relationship with alcohol won't happen overnight, and you can use a slip to learn about yourself. You are running a marathon here, not a sprint! And if you trip and fall on mile sixteen, would you stay down and give up? Would you sulk and tell yourself you'll try to run the race again next year? Or will you get up and keep going and finish the race? Don't let a misstep devastate the entire learning experience. I don't care that you slipped—I care what you do next. Success doesn't mean never failing. True success means getting back up again when you do. Again and again and again. I love a Japanese proverb about falling down: Fall down seven times, get up eight.

If things haven't gone exactly as you planned, it's okay. You can learn a lot from your missteps: what triggers you, what emotions need to be processed in healthy ways, and where the false romance of alcohol still holds strong. You can also learn if alcohol feels worth it or is even satiating (spoiler alert: it usually doesn't and isn't). All these points help you create a better journey going forward. You're making progress just by reading this book. You're already wildly successful. Haven't had a slip or wobble? Keep going strong!

WEEK 3 MOCKTAIL

GREEN SMOOTHIE

I love to drink a green smoothie every day, to sneak more veggies into my life. The avocado makes it creamy and helps blend the greens. You can swap in kale or add frozen mango. Feel free to experiment and find the combination that's most delicious to you.

MAKES 3 SERVINGS

- 1 banana, peeled and sliced
- 1 avocado, halved, pitted, peeled, and sliced
- 1 apple, cored and sliced
- 115g spinach
- 1 tablespoon ground flax seed
- 1 teaspoon turmeric
- 1.2l water (or use coconut water or plant-based milk)

Put the banana, avocado, apple, spinach, ground flax seed, turmeric, and water in a blender and blend on high for 3 minutes. I drink one-third of the smoothie right away, then pour the rest in a mason jar to save in the refrigerator for later.

YOUR JOURNALING HOMEWORK

This week, we're going to start the powerful practice of visualization. Get your journal, put on some meditation music, sit down, and relax. Take four long, deep breaths. Imagine it's a year from today. You kept going on your alcohol-free journey and don't miss drinking a bit. Everything in your life has improved, including a surge of confidence and a belief that anything is possible.

You feel incredible in your skin, love moving your body, and are fitter and healthier than you've ever been. You love to take care of yourself. You appreciate your body so much, its strength and stamina, and are filled with energy to take on your wildest dreams.

What does this look like to you? Think of three imaginative ways you take better care of your health. Are you a long-distance runner? A yoga teacher or enthusiast? What does your relationship to healthy foods look like? What do you eat? Do you cook more? Let your imagination have fun.

At the end of your visualization, journal about what you saw. Can you see how the lifestyle you're embarking on could lead you to your dream goals? In contrast, do you think drinking alcohol could lead you there?

Navigate Your Social Life

Woohoo! It's week 4, and you're doing amazing! I'm impressed and inspired by your commitment to self-discovery. You're becoming stronger, braver, and more intuitive than you've ever been. And that newfound confidence and self-esteem will serve you tremendously, because it's time to take this challenge out into your public life. While it may seem easier to hole up for your two-month break, it's part of your skill-building and limiting beliefs-debunking to get out there and socialize!

The first thing you need to realize is this: being alcohol-free isn't embarrassing. I know it can be nerve-racking to be asked about your decision not to drink. Most of us worry about what other people think of us and what stories they are making up in their heads. We're human, after all. But giving up alcohol isn't you admitting to some huge weakness—it doesn't say anything about you, your personality, or your willpower. All it says is that you're open to discovering what life looks like without hangovers and that you want to see what you're capable of without a toxic beverage in your life.

Not drinking alcohol is one of the healthiest things you could do, physically, mentally, and emotionally. To think that not drinking signals a problem rather than being a huge advantage is a tired old paradigm. Lay it to bed and pick up the bravado to believe you're here because your soul tapped you to discover your fullest potential. You are made for more than drinking every weekend. You're lucky.

COME UP WITH YOUR PERFECT ONE-LINER

When you get offered a drink or someone asks if you'd like one, I want you to tap into that confident spirit that makes you feel like a queen. You'll also feel more comfortable when you have a simple and easy response to explain why you're not drinking. I tell people I don't drink and don't think twice about it, but this might only work for people you've never met before, who don't know you as anything other than a nondrinker. For others, simply go with, "Thanks, I'm great" (no one can argue with you when you're doing great), "Yes, I'd love a sparkling water," or "I feel so much healthier without it. Thanks, though!" Or you could say you're doing a challenge to see how your life or health will improve without alcohol. You might be amazed at how well people respond to honesty and bravery. It sounds pretty cool and may pique others' interests.

You also don't owe anyone your story. You don't have to share the deeper ins and outs of your insecurities or internal stress with anyone if you don't want to, especially not a random acquaintance at a party. What feels comfortable to you will be unique and may vary over time. In the beginning, some people feel safer offering an excuse. One of my clients used early work mornings and health detoxes to say, "No, thank you." It's okay to stumble a little at first. One day, your answer will come effortlessly, and you may come to love the opportunity to share with others why you don't drink and the beautiful life you've found without alcohol. There is a lot of power in saying, "I don't drink." And if people demand to know why, especially rudely, you can flip the question back at them and ask, "Why do you drink?"

NOBODY CARES . . . UNLESS THEY DO

My clients are often pleasantly surprised to learn that most people don't care whether you're drinking or not. We make it out to be such a huge deal in our minds, but half the people around you won't even notice. Some people will be genuinely curious and politely ask a lot of questions. They've probably thought about doing something like this before, and you're becoming an inspiration and a role model for them. It would have rocked my world to see people at a party not drinking a few years ago. It would have shattered my preconceived notion that you have to drink socially. When someone asks curiously, remember that this is bigger than you. The person is probably asking for his or her own benefit and not trying to make you feel small. You're giving permission to question the role of alcohol in that person's life too. You have no idea what doors or windows you're opening in other people's mindsets.

And if people make you feel small or silly for doing something like this or belittling you by saying how much control they feel around alcohol? They're not talking about you at all. This is called deflecting. They're deflecting from the fact that they, too, have doubts and insecurities around their own drinking patterns. You're threatening them and their worldview and holding up a mirror to their habits. They might even feel judged because your drinking habits were previously similar to theirs. We emulate the five people we're closest to, and it's no coincidence that your friends are drinkers too.[1] They might even try to goad you into drinking simply because it's embarrassing to drink alone, and hence the reason many drinkers encourage others to drink. Hell, I certainly did when I was hosting. Put on your psychologist hat and try to understand the motivations behind other people's actions instead of making it mean something about you. It usually doesn't. They're reacting to you through the lens of their own drinking pattern. And last, remember that this isn't high school anymore. No one has the power to make you feel dumb because you aren't drinking a type of beverage. Laugh off peer pressure and let yourself feel like the radiant goddess that you are.

PICTURE THE ALTERNATIVE

There will be a lot of firsts on this journey. Your first night out. Your first dinner party. Your first wedding. Your first networking event. Places where most people are drinking around you, but you're not. The last thing you want to do is have a pity party for yourself. This is a chance to experience the event with all your senses, make new insights, and feel amazing the next day. You get to laugh authentically with your friends, dance, and wake up early the next day. One of my favorite tools to shift one's mindset from FOMO to JOMO is called *picture the alternative.*

Picturing the alternative means taking off the rose-tinted glasses and giving yourself a mental play-by-play of how drinking actually feels—not the romanticized version, the real one. All the mental gymnastics, all the chatter, all the times you betrayed your intentions, and even all the times you wanted more but stopped and felt disappointed. So much mental space given to a fermented liquid. When you go alcohol-free to an event, you'll notice that the internal chatter is gone.

The next time you're faced with a situation in which you would have been drinking previously, picture what the night would look like for you if you decided to drink. Would it be fun to have a few glasses of wine and then get coaxed into shots of tequila and wake up on a stranger's couch, with a rocking headache? Even if that's not how it would play out, how would you feel after a few drinks? Vibrant and energetic? How would you sleep that night? Soundly and deeply? How would you feel in the morning? Proud and accomplished? I'm guessing not, and you'd likely feel way more negative feelings than positive ones. I want you to continue to think about situations and social engagements you encounter and envision how the night would have gone for you if you had drunk. This exercise also works well for nights you don't go out because it helps you identify the contrast in your life. Now that you're not drinking, you're not succumbing to all the mental anguish, broken promises, bad experiences, and lost afternoons, evenings, and mornings.

SOCIALIZING TIPS

Now that you have the mindset tool to feel lucky that you're not drinking socially, let's dive into some other helpful tips. If you've ever felt socially awkward before, welcome to the club. As I've mentioned, I'm an introvert and love authentically connecting with a few people at a time, but put me in a huge room of networkers, and you might see me sneak off to the bathroom a few times. Kidding, but not really. I don't think you need to be an introvert to feel social anxiety in large groups of people you don't know. Socializing with people you just met or hardly know is awkward, for everyone involved! Most people hate small talk. The first five to fifteen minutes of a social event can be weird, but trust that you'll ease into it.

One thing on your side is your ability to truly connect with others. Let yourself listen more and ask questions. It takes the attention off of you and builds stronger connections. People appreciate it when others are genuinely interested in their lives. One of my clients started to realize how inauthentic she was to her true personality when she drank, because she was loud and disinterested in other people. Bring the real you and watch what happens. You have a great capacity for deep and meaningful conversations that may foster much deeper relationships with the people you care about. You're building your socializing muscle, which you have to flex and practice with.

Each time you socialize alcohol-free, allow yourself to visualize how amazing you'll feel in the morning. In essence, you get to have your cake and eat it too. You can socialize and still feel fresh, energetic, and happy the next day. You get to do so much more, not less. It might also help to juxtapose your evening and subsequent morning with those of the people around you who are drinking. They might look merry at the party, but everyone around you with a drink in their hand won't wake up as fresh and happy as you will. Feel free to gloat a little, smug in the knowledge that you're putting your well-being first.

HOW TO MAKE LIKE-MINDED FRIENDS

Here's where things get really exciting. A whole world of people is out there who are living their best lives without alcohol, who will push you to keep growing and go after the dreams on your heart. This lifestyle offers you the chance to meet a lot of new friends, because most people are hungry to see their new lifestyle reflected in others! And there's a lot going on in the alcohol-free space.

One of the best places to start your search is on meetup. com. See if there are any alcohol-free social groups in your area. Try searching the keywords *sober* or *alcohol-free*. Most big cities have a few options. These groups get together and do things like go on hikes, do yoga, or get brunch. And if you don't see one in your city, could you form one yourself? Remember: being alcohol-free makes you brave! Another great option if you live in a big city is to see if there's a mocktail bar in your area. Places like New York, San Francisco, Los Angeles, Denver, London, and Dublin have mocktail bars and many more cities have pop-ups and events.

You also can make friends online. I've met a lot of dear sisters in my life who started out as online friends and morphed into some of my nearest and dearest. You can start on Instagram and engage on alcohol-free accounts (you can find me at @euphoric.af) and reach out to people. Facebook also has tons of private groups you can join, with thousands of members; some are bound to live in your area. We'll regularly ask members in the Euphoric Facebook group where they live, so they can start connecting with each other. And lastly, group coaching is one of my favorite ways to become quickly and deeply connected with other women. The Become Euphoric™ Group Coaching program is offered a few times a year, and the connections women have made there astound me.

You also don't have to restrict your search solely by what's alcohol-free. Many growth-oriented spaces are filled with people trying to live their healthiest and best lives. Look into yoga groups, hiking meetups, and personal growth conferences or spiritual events. I meet nondrinkers everywhere I go because

I'm obsessed with personal growth. Many people equally obsessed with living the life of their dreams hardly have time for alcohol, or drink so infrequently it's irrelevant.

The point is, when you surround yourself with friends who are launching their own businesses, writing books, running marathons, traveling the world, or living their best wellness or spiritual lifestyle, going to the bars every weekend stops being the norm. The new norm inspires you and gives you something to aspire to. And if you're competitive by nature, there's no better way to radically change your life than by hanging out with other go-getters.

YOUR JOURNALING HOMEWORK

Go back to your journal entry from week 1 and revisit the top reasons you like to drink. Now that you've been experiencing life alcohol-free for almost four weeks, you probably have a lot of alternative evidence to prove those beliefs wrong. Take each belief and ask yourself: Is it scientifically true? Is it fundamentally true no matter what? Is it true for all people? Does it empower me or disempower me? And can you find alternative evidence to prove the opposite of each statement?

Some of the reasons why I used to like to drink were: Drinking makes me confident while socializing, drinking increases my social life, drinking reduces stress, drinking relaxes me, drinking numbs pain, drinking is fun, and drinking is sophisticated.

- *Drinking reduces stress.* If reducing stress means putting your head in the sand for a while, then sure. Drinking merely took me out of my mind for a while. Everything I was stressed about was still there in the morning and compounded by a headache or hangover. I had more ruminating and racing thoughts. Drinking also made me feel less capable of handling my life. It added more stress and worries, not less.

- *Drinking is fun.* Drinking might seem fun in the moment, but how much can that be attributed to drinking versus the fun situation I was in? I always drank at social occasions, so did the alcohol make it fun, or was it fun because I enjoy hanging out, laughing with, and talking with my friends? Sometimes it seemed like staying in and watching a movie was fun with some wine. But halfway through the movie, I'd stop being interested and get sidetracked by social media. Sounds pretty dull to me.

Keep these new beliefs handy and be patient about the process. Your old beliefs took thirty-plus years to form around alcohol. Deconstructing them can take time and effort, but it's so worth it.

WEEK 4 MOCKTAIL

Try a Kin Euphorics, Saint Ivy Moscow Mule, Gruvi Dry Secco, Curious Elixirs, or Surreal Brewing nonalcoholic beer!

Get Mindful and Embody Self-Love

You're doing something huge: You are living life fully alive. You are experiencing the full breadth of your emotions without numbing them. This is a chance to get to know yourself and become present and deeply aware of your inner desires and needs. This week, we'll take a look at what your emotions are telling you and how to lean in and cultivate mindful presence. Feeling unmasked or a little raw at this point is normal. Being able to feel means you're able to heal your inner landscape and change the way you think and feel in the future. Alcohol allows you to numb the uncomfortable, the boring, the stressful, the sad, pushing these emotions further down into your psyche. But you can't selectively numb the bad and not numb the good as well. Feeling happier isn't a matter of blocking your negative emotions, but rather processing them.

●　●　●

IDENTIFY AND EXPRESS YOUR FEELINGS

I love to think of emotions as barometers, or teachers that help us learn where we need to make shifts in our lives. For example, feeling resentment at your partner isn't something you have to swallow. It's a sign that things need to change, vulnerable conversations need to be had, or boundaries need to be put up. When we're used to numbing our emotions, sometimes it's hard to even know what we feel! There are four base emotions: anger, sadness, joy, and fear.[1] The subtler ones are often mixtures of these. For example, nostalgia is a mix of joy and sadness. Stress is a mix of anger and fear. Going alcohol-free helped me pay attention to my emotions. I learned how to better handle uncomfortable feelings and develop new outlets of expression for them, instead of keeping them pent up. This process takes a lot of mindfulness.

From a young age, we're taught not to feel our emotions. *Stop crying. Calm down. Don't get too excited.* And so our emotions grow and fester inside of us. Every time I felt insecure and reached for a drink, I escaped that feeling and didn't learn how to work through it. I didn't use any tools to talk back to my inner critic or soothe my inner child, who was feeling the insecurity. If I'd had tools to use, the next time I felt insecure at a party, I would've made progress in dealing with that uncomfortable emotion, perhaps even to the point of surpassing it. Instead of creating a life of emotional progress, drinking stunts us emotionally.

Life isn't going to be rosy all the time. It comes with uncomfortable feelings that you're meant to work through, even when it feels stupid to indulge the feeling. Early in my alcohol-free journey, I remember a time I went to a party with my sister's running friends. I was excited to share with them how I'd stopped drinking and had all these fun alcohol-free drinks to share. No one asked, and no one cared. I felt so stupid. It reminded me of feeling that way when I was a child, doing something I thought would get me love and attention only to realize that it's not that special, which in turn made me feel like *I* wasn't that special. But instead of telling myself I was acting silly and to move on, I allowed myself to express my disappointment and sadness. I took a bath that night with a slow Florence + The Machine playlist and cried. It only lasted about ten minutes, but I felt much better afterward. I honored my feelings and didn't make myself feel even more dumb for having them.

My clients are rock stars in developing new methods to express their emotions. When Laura was feeling restless at 7:00 p.m., she injected some wonder and exploration into her life by going for a walk at sunset. When Sara felt stressed and angry about her job, she used a smash ball (those heavy workout balls) to throw and vent her anger from her body through the ball to the ground. If Andrea felt somewhat exposed and fearful, she knew she needed to work through her body with yoga and dance. Alex felt crazy adrenaline after work, so she incorporated meditation rituals to release her natural calm. Mike turned to meditation and prayer. When you express your emotions, you feel relief.

You're not supposed to feel angry, stressed, and resentful all the time. Those emotions are popping up to tell you that you need to make changes in your life. They're showing you how to notice when something is wrong and not aligned with what you really want. And you can always use the tool of journaling to get clarity. Journaling helps you connect with what's underneath the emotion. A few of my clients noticed a lot of negative emotions around their work. Instead of ignoring this and trudging through the slog, as many of us do with our careers, they're planning moves and exciting new opportunities.

If you're pissed off, resentful, frustrated, or stressed, only you can make the changes in your life or circumstances to address these emotions. You might need to have honest conversations or put up new boundaries. And don't fret—this isn't an all-or-nothing situation. In week 7, I'll teach you how to make changes via baby steps.

Drinking over your feelings tells your inner self that it's not okay to experience your full breadth of emotions. What you don't feel, you can't learn from. Sometimes, it's through the hardest challenges and greatest adversities that people discover what they're meant to do. You're feeling your emotions for a reason. Use this week to lean in, journal through, and express them in new ways.

NEGATIVE THOUGHTS

While your emotions are sensations that your body is meant to process, you'll also have to come to terms with your thoughts. Not all of them are worth listening to. Every one of us has an inner critic that tells us we're ultimately not good enough in some way: not smart enough, not capable enough, not pretty enough, not loveable enough. The inner critic is the voice of the ego, the overly protective and fearful part of us that's trying to survive, not thrive. The inner critic is like an overly protective grandma; if she had it her way, you'd never leave the house and try anything new. The voice tries to protect you from pain and disappointment, often by being the harshest person you know. For example, when a woman berates herself in front of the mirror and tells herself she's fat, that's her inner critic hurting her first, before the outside world gets the chance.

My inner critic told me I was doomed to repeat my mistakes with drinking forever (safer to remove any hope). It told me that I couldn't write a book. That I couldn't launch a business. That I couldn't make new friends. That I had a weird-looking face. That I'm not relatable or even likeable. That I'm incapable of success. And because we're not taught how to manage our thoughts in healthy ways, I accepted this voice as truth. I didn't realize how universal the inner critic was—and that I am not my thoughts.

As I shared earlier, scientists have found that we have around sixty thousand unique thoughts a day; 95 percent of these thoughts are repeat thoughts from the previous day, and 80 percent are negative.[2] The danger lies in getting carried away in the thoughts and believing them as ultimate truth. As you get mindful this week, you'll learn how to manage your critical thoughts, so you can free yourself from the limiting stories they're telling you. When you start to see your inner critic as something outside of you, separate from your higher consciousness, you can better discern which voice to listen to.

Learning more about the negative thoughts that chatter away in your brain helps you disengage from the story. In *Change Your Brain, Change Your Life,* neuroscientist Daniel Amen, MD, shows us that our negative thoughts aren't unique to us—they follow patterns that all humans fall into.[3] For example, *all-or-nothing thoughts* means we fall into the trap of thinking everything has to be perfect to be good, and if it's not perfect, it's a failure. A classic example is the way many people approach diet plans with a perfectionist's attitude: either I do it perfectly, or I quit. If I eat some cake at a birthday party, I might as well gorge on pizza later too. With alcohol, this kind of thinking is dangerous. Slipping once isn't a reason to start drinking again. Life isn't all-or-nothing—it's about making progress.

Another example of negative thoughts is *blame thoughts*, where you blame other people for problems instead of taking responsibility. Take an average marital spat: "It's your fault I dropped the plate because you were rushing me." These thoughts are self-defeating because they make you the victim in a world you can't control. They make you feel powerless to change your behaviors and situation because you don't think you're responsible. For example, thinking that this eight-week challenge is hard because your partner or friends drink is a blame thought. In reality, changing your life for the better has nothing to do with your partner's or friends' habits, and blaming them absolves you of responsibility.

You don't have to believe the story your inner critic tells you. You can stop, question the thought's validity, and break through its limiting power over you. And make sure you have compassion for yourself. We'd never talk to our friends or kids the way we often do to ourselves. Another great technique to use when you're having negative thoughts is the emotional freedom technique or tapping. Similar to the concept of acupressure, tapping is a technique you can do yourself, by tapping meridian points on your head and chest while expressing your emotions and then turning them around with positive affirmations to help soothe yourself. When I walk my clients through this, we tap on these meridian points, express any negative feelings, and turn them around with gentler, more compassionate thoughts, such as *I'm doing the best I can, I'm learning, I'm an infinite being, I'm doing soulful work.* Check out www.euphoricaf.com/book-bonus to see it in action and do it yourself.

THE GIFT OF GRATITUDE

The absolute fastest way to turn around negative thoughts is to change your focus. Whatever we focus on expands in our minds. You can choose to focus on things that are going well and feel thankful. Gratitude has little to do with your mood, whether you've had a good day, how much is in your bank account, or how successful you think you are. Gratitude isn't a feeling only lucky people have—it's something that needs to be practiced. There are people on this planet who'd give anything to have the things and lifestyle you have. Did you wake up in bed today? Did you have a delicious breakfast that nourishes your body? Can you safely go to work or school because your country isn't in a civil war? Are you surrounded by loved ones, if even a furry one?

Go ahead: stop right now and write down ten things you're grateful for that happened within the past twenty-four hours. I like limiting my list to smaller things instead of constantly expressing gratitude for big things, because it helps me recognize smaller blessings that are happening around me all the time. While I could list my gratitude for dog's or my husband's love every single day, I try to remember how nice it was to have a deep conversation with my husband, feel the sun hit my face on a chilly day, or hear an encouraging comment from a friend. If you did this every day, it would fundamentally make you a happier person, who's always looking for the good in the world.

Sometimes I'll feel such a strong wave of gratitude hit me that tears well up in my eyes, and I feel struck by pure grace and love. I feel grateful for the miracle of being alive in this time and place. Grateful for the mystery and beauty of living in an abundant, magical universe. Grateful for the fact that

I've woken up to the magnitude of my life and its infinite possibilities. Trust me—I never had moments like this after drinking. Instead, I was jealous, petty, and judgmental of others. I played small and didn't let myself dream. The sublime beauty of this world was lost on me.

You, too, are awakening. It's not every day that people wake up and know they're destined for more. It's not every day that people listen to that voice of intuition and stop settling for less. Most people don't know their deeper why. They also work in unfulfilling careers, feel unhealthy, have poor social connections, and live by society's expectations of them, not their own. Yet you are here, forming a deep communion with your deepest inner wishes for yourself, which will serve you for the rest of your life. Let yourself be grateful and happy you get this second chance at your dream life. It won't be unicorns and butterflies all the time, but you have the tools to see a greater perspective and allow your gratitude practice to create feelings of appreciation. However, gratitude doesn't merely keep you positive. Studies show that gratitude practices predict better cardiovascular health, lower inflammation in the body, and lower stress hormones.[4] It does your mind and body good.

CULTIVATE MINDFULNESS

This entire experience has been an exercise in mindfulness. Instead of functioning on autopilot and getting mindless each time you reach for a drink, you've been unearthing the reasons behind your drive to drink and finding what will fulfill and grow you instead. You're learning how to sit with your feelings and thoughts instead of getting caught up with them. You're allowing yourself to be present to the unfolding of life, present to every mundane yet beautiful moment.

If you don't have a formal mindfulness practice, now is the perfect time to introduce one. Great spiritual teachers say that practices such a prayer, contemplation, meditation, or just sitting or walking in silence can help us connect to our truest purpose. A mindfulness practice helps you sort out distractions and competing voices and get to the core of your higher self. Meditation is also known for its health benefits. It helps reduce stress and the underlying causes that develop heart disease. It also helps reduce anxiety and promotes a sense of mental wellness. It helps you become more self-aware (and identify your inner critic) and improves self-esteem.[5]

I've been meditating for years now and like to change up my practice. Sometimes I'll do breathwork or a guided visualization, or I'll focus on one word or phrase. It's great to meditate in the morning, on your lunch break, or anytime you need to center yourself and step off the hamster wheel of life.

Guided meditations can be the easiest way to get started, and tons of free ones are out there. I use the app Insight Timer, which is filled with thousands of guided or instrumental mediations. If meditating is something you want to cultivate in your life, next week I'll show you how to find extra time in your schedule for some personal growth activities. You don't have to strive for perfection—just try your best. Meditating might not be something you care to incorporate, and that's okay too. Many other practices can help you become more mindful and aware of your inner landscape: doing yoga, walking in nature, being in the moment when you're doing the dishes, and simply looking around yourself and taking deep breaths and pauses in your daily life.

* * *

EMBODYING SELF-LOVE

In part II, I shared how much I missed the mark on truly loving and taking care of myself when I didn't regard future me as worth taking care of. *Oh well, I'll sleep it off,* I'd think when I knew I was drinking too much. Not being able to trust myself also eroded my belief that I was even capable or worthy of such love. My thoughts, feelings, and behaviors all coalesced to create a negative spiral. By expressing your emotions, managing your thoughts, and taking care of yourself on a whole new level, your spiral goes upward, as does your self-worth. You're showing up every day and trying to do the things that make you the person you want to be. This intentionality shifts your self-esteem. You start believing you're capable of much more than you ever believed. You start trusting yourself again, and that newfound trust and confidence trickles into other areas of your life.

When you show up and try to do the things that will make you a better person, you become a better person. When you do it at this level of introspection, it's harder for you to keep ignoring what you aspire to be and how you do want to be remembered in this life. Expressing your emotions and managing your critical thoughts means you give yourself more compassion and love. When we feel bad, we often make ourselves feel wrong for feeling bad. It's like an emotion stacked on an emotion. You don't have to feel guilty or ashamed for the way you feel. Express yourself fully, then let it go. When a thought tells you you'll never make it, you don't have to accept that at face value.

Embodying self-love is also living life according to your deepest values. My top values include freedom, purpose, growth, happiness, abundance, confidence, creativity, health, and connection. Your values might be different, and that's part of what makes each of us unique. When I'm living in alignment with these values, I feel fulfilled and thriving. When I'm misaligned, it's painful because I'm being incongruent with my intrinsic self. If I reflect on how the drinking version of me honored these values, I can't say that she did. I valued health, yet I purposely made myself feel unwell every weekend. I valued happiness, yet I was drinking a beverage that alters your brain chemistry to make you feel more depressed and apathetic. I valued authenticity and connection, yet I used alcohol as an artificial crutch to connect with others.

Sit for a moment and think about your top five values. Which version of you—drinking or alcohol-free—allows you to live in congruence with them? Living life fully aligned with your values creates harmony and peace of mind.

WEEK 5 MOCKTAIL

GUAVA ROSE

Embody even more self-love this week with this gorgeous rose mocktail.

MAKES 1 SERVING

- 90ml rose tea, steeped
- 120ml guava nectar or juice
- 1.5 tablespoons rose water
- 1 teaspoon grenadine, for color
- Ice
- Sparkling water, to taste

Put the rose tea, guava nectar, rose water, and grenadine in a cocktail shaker with ice and shake vigorously. Pour the mixture into a glass with ice. Top with sparkling water to your liking.

YOUR JOURNALING HOMEWORK

Your ability to go deep and create this level of insight in your life is nothing short of remarkable. This week, use the following reflections to go even deeper:

- Think of ways to express your emotions, and then do them this week! For example, when you feel angry, you can punch a pillow or do a high-intensity interval workout. When you feel sad, you can take a bath, cry, and treat yourself like a child that needs comfort and reassurance.
- What are you grateful for this week? Does focusing on it change your mood or perspective?
- How did drinking affect your self-esteem and self-love? Do you see a shift since you've been alcohol-free? What does self-love mean to you today?
- What are your top five values? Which version of you—drinking or alcohol-free—allows you to live in congruence with them?
- What's one mindfulness practice you'd like to incorporate into your life?

Find Pure and Utter Happiness

Now that you're taking care of your basic emotions without using alcohol to cope, you're building a strong emotional foundation and supporting your mental well-being. It's like the gaps are filled, and you can layer on the good stuff to design a life you love. This week is all about incorporating rituals and routines into your daily life, to help you feel happier. You can call it the art of daily living. We'll also go over the top human needs and ways to get extra creative in meeting those needs without a drink.

DESIGN A MORNING ROUTINE YOU LOVE

As I shared in part I, you're going to start falling in love with your mornings. No more waking up on the wrong side of the bed, frazzled and distraught, barely able to keep up with your life. Now that you're getting the hang of this, it's time to construct a morning routine, which come in all shapes and sizes. The basic idea is that you wake up a little earlier than you have to, so you can prioritize the activities that make you feel mentally and physically amazing. It's also the best opportunity to have some "me time," before anyone else in the house and responsibilities awaken. Whatever you want to prioritize in your life, fit it in here. Then you'll feel a sense of peace, calm, and accomplishment before the chaos of the day starts. The most successful people in the world credit their morning routines for allowing them to be on top of their game.

First up, plan what you want to do during this time. Here's a bank of activities you could choose from: reading personal growth books, journaling, meditating, visualizing your dream life, saying or writing affirmations, creative writing, gratitude journaling, working on a side passion project, exercising, preparing healthy foods for the day, anointing yourself with oils and adorning yourself with makeup, and so on. The ideas are endless. Once you have a plan, set your alarm!

At first, try waking up thirty minutes earlier. I'll either wake up an hour earlier during the spring and summer months and sometimes just twenty minutes earlier during colder months. If you have trouble getting out of bed in the morning, here are some tips:

- Set your alarm on the far side of the bedroom, so you're forced to jump out of bed when it goes off. Don't go back to bed or hit snooze.
- Cuddle your dog or cat. This will immediately help you feel more comfort, especially since you just left your warm covers.
- Go to the bathroom and brush your teeth. Splash some water on your face.
- Drink a tall glass of water.

- If you drink coffee or tea, set the pot to brew
  automatically, so you can anticipate a hot drink
  right away.

Make sure you don't check your phone or emails during
your morning routine. It's not the time to be in reactive mode.
This is your proactive mode. Try your morning routine for at
least two weeks and see if your mood and sense of accomplishment is affected for the rest of the day. If you want to live a life
you love, you have to do things differently in your day. A morning routine also gives you a lot of intentional time to yourself,
which will give you clarity and insights into your bigger passions and dreams.

EVENING ROUTINE AND OTHER RITUALS

Evening routines can have a lot less structure than morning
ones because you'll have different things and events to manage. But it's nice to have a routine for your normal nights in.
My evening routine is drawn from a bank of these activities:
taking a bath, brushing my skin, practicing yin yoga, reading,
journaling, doing guided meditations or visualizations, and a
simple ritual of taking care of my face and teeth. Obviously,
not all evenings can be this expansive because you might be
doing other fun life activities, like date night, hanging with
friends, taking care of kids, or watching a movie. But when
nothing else is going on, I like to retire to my bedroom early
and have some me time.

You can play around with the other times of your day that
are usually swept into the chaos and find moments of peace
and quiet there too. For example, take an actual break for
lunch and go for a walk or read. Take more frequent breaks

from your desk and stretch, meditate, or get a healthy snack. Listen to uplifting music or motivating podcasts on your commute. Regularly incorporate the things that bring you the most joy into your every day. Do something nice for yourself— you deserve it!

MEET YOUR NEEDS IN CREATIVE WAYS

As you continue to decipher your needs, you'll experiment with meeting them in creative new ways. Abraham Maslow first defined the top human needs in the 1940s, and a few different models have followed. My favorite way of explaining our common needs comes from Tony Robbins. The six top needs are: certainty, uncertainty, significance, love and connection, growth, and contribution.[1] I'll show you how these needs were being poorly met with alcohol and then give you ideas to be creative with how you meet them today.

Certainty pertains to our need to feel safe and secure, have our basic needs met, feel comforted, and have predictable routines. Drinking plays a role here when we use it to retreat to a predictable comfort zone or chill out. This often happens after a hard or stressful day. The need for *uncertainty* is the opposite. It's the human need for variety and adventure. It's about changing your state of being, experiencing new things, having unknowns, and enjoying a sense of fun. Drinking is all about changing your state and inviting in a sense of an unknown risk. It's used to feel wild, let loose, lose your inhibitions, and feel like you're taking a risk. Like when it's Friday night, and you're ready to celebrate.

Significance is about feeling important. People seek significance through recognition from others. It's about feeling special and having achievements, accolades, reputation, or status.

Drinking can be about significance when you use it to show off your status or sophistication, for example, with wine cellars, trips to Bordeaux, and "glamorous" martinis. Status could even be about how "bad" you are—for example, drinking like a guy, staying up late, playing drinking games.

Love and connection are about our deep need to feel connected with something or someone. We all need to feel loved and in union with others. When drinking socially, alcohol can be misguidedly used to meet the need for connection or thinking that you're bonding over booze.

These first four needs are called "needs of the personality," whereas the last two are "needs of the spirit" and bring more long-lasting joy and fulfillment.[2] *Growth* is our birthright. As I stated earlier in the book, everything in the universe is either growing or dying. Growth governs our needs to progress in our understanding, evolution, and capacity. We can grow ourselves emotionally, intellectually, physically, and spiritually. *Contribution* is all about spiritual fulfilment. It pertains to our need to give back, help others, make an impact, be the difference, and support others. Alcohol has little to do with the last two needs and is more involved with the four needs of the personality. As you can see, the first four needs can be met in healthy or unhealthy ways.

It's not wrong to have these needs. You just have to ask yourself if alcohol was meeting them and get creative about what you can intentionally do to get the feelings you desire. For example, at one point or another, many of my clients realize they have a need for uncertainty and feeling wild. You do all the right things when you don't drink, such as make healthy choices and be productive, and the urge to rebel can suddenly hit you. This isn't a bad thing. I tell my clients to let out their inner wild woman, who needs to feel a sense of adventure, risk, and newness. One of my favorite ways to meet this need is to jump into a cold body of water. I do this a few times a year, and there's nothing like it. When I do it, I feel like a badass—pure, raw power like an animal. Other ideas include:

- Go on a steep, challenging hike or an indoor mountain climb.
- Do a naked full-moon ritual.
- Sing at the top of your lungs at karaoke (or in your car).
- Dance your heart out on a stage (or in a living room). Is there anything crazier or more thrilling than signing or dancing full out while completely sober? It's actually pretty wild.

You could even do something simple for yourself. Leave the house or work on a Tuesday afternoon and go peruse your favorite shop or see a matinee. All these activities give you a sense of uncertainty.

In the opposite vein, if I want comfort, my faves include yin yoga, a holiday movie, tea, morning and evening routines, and tasty vegan food. You can meet your need for significance by indulging in something glamourous, like a five-course chef tasting menu or dressing up and going to the opera. You could become an expert in alcohol-free drinks and pairings. You could become an entrepreneur or expert in your field. And you can tap into your inner rebel by doing what most people won't: be alcohol-free. I meet my need for love and connection by being a part of sister circles and mastermind groups. I have date nights with my husband and start deep conversations. I go on trips with my parents or babysit my niece and nephew.

Alcohol doesn't contribute to the needs of the spirit, which is the reason drinking feels unfulfilling at the end of the day. Meeting your need for growth could look like constant personal exploration, self-discovery, learning, coaching, courses, making progress, and so on. Contribution is about giving back: Teaching what you've learned. Helping the past version of you. Volunteering. Raising money for charity.

As you can see, with any of these ideas, you're an active player and agent in creating your own happiness. Don't give it away to chance.

FEEL GOOD ORGANICALLY

By incorporating routines and creative ways to meet your needs, you'll drastically increase the amount of positive emotions you experience on a daily basis. And let's not forget: the very act of being alcohol-free allows your neurochemistry to rebalance. Being a drinker means you have lowered levels of dopamine, serotonin, and GABA, and heightened levels of cortisol, adrenaline, and dynorphin coursing through your brain. As a drinker, I often felt on edge, low, and in need of relief. And how often do we drink because we want to "take the edge off"? How paradoxical that it's drinking that puts us "on edge" in the first place.

I spent time drinking because I thought I enjoyed the buzz. But that artificial buzz masks your natural buzz. Our bodies enable us to tap into natural buzzes all on their own. You feel it when you have a belly laugh with your friend. You feel it when you do something that scares you, yet you go for it anyway. You feel it when you're outside in a forest. You feel it when you dance and sing. You feel it when you stargaze. You feel it when you find something you're so passionate about, you lose track of time. This is being euphoric.

You won't feel happy all the time, but that's not the point. The point is to feel all your feelings and learn from them. Happiness means doing your part. Working on yourself, taking care of your body and mental health, and incorporating practices into your life—like a morning routine, gratitude practice, intentional connection, goal setting, and self-reflection—that change your state in a healing way. It means expressing your emotions and intentionally overriding your negative thoughts or inner critic with new, positive beliefs. It also means making shifts where shifts need to be made. I don't feel happy 100 percent of the time. Instead of numbing my bad feelings, I let myself feel them, cry, journal, and reflect. They don't last long, because I'm taking the steps to uncover and resolve the underlying issues. This work isn't always easy, and it lasts your whole life. But it's worth it, and you deserve it.

Happiness also comes from expressing your desires and feeling passionate about what you do. Next week, we'll dive deeper into trying new things, finding your passions, and letting yourself dream.

WEEK 6 MOCKTAIL

SPICY GRAPEFRUIT

I love pink drinks. They make me happy.

MAKES 1 SERVING

- Juice of one large grapefruit
- Juice of half a lemon
- 1 teaspoon grenadine
- 6 slices jalapeño or serrano pepper
- Ice

Put the grapefruit juice, lemon juice, grenadine, and three jalapeño slices in a shaker with ice and shake vigorously. Pour the mixture in a short glass with ice and garnish with three jalapeño slices.

YOUR JOURNALING HOMEWORK

Find a day this week to do what brings you the most joy. Write down a plan for the most perfect relaxing day.

I'd start my day with a big cup of coffee on my patio, along with my journal and a good book. I'd spend the early morning reading and writing. Then I'd love to go exploring, whether walking through a farmers market or going on a new hiking trail with my hubby and dog. For dinner, I'd go to a hip restaurant I've been wanting to try. And my perfect day would end with enough time for a relaxing bath and more reading before bed. It's simple, doable, and pure joy to me.

Use today as a test pilot for what you want to infuse into your every day.

Create Your Dream Life

With all the time, clarity, energy, and joy that becomes available to you when you're alcohol-free, you're able to live a new life. Filled with new passions, hobbies, and experiences. This week, we'll explore your interests, try new things, and allow new experiences to open the door to your creativity and greater purpose.

I did things that were totally out of my norm. The momentum of getting out of my comfort zone and not drinking, plus all that extra free time I gained, pushed me forward into new territories and activities. Being more playful and exploratory reminded me of being a kid. There's a reason you've always wanted to try tango dancing or planting a garden. It's time to explore!

EXPLORE YOUR INTERESTS

While it can be hard to imagine how going to a new class or trying a new activity could change your life, hear me out on this. It helps you broaden your perspective and adds new skills that expand your identity. Who knows? Those very skills could apply later, when you define your purpose. Just the skill of putting yourself out there and trying something as a beginner broadens your mind. It's easy to say *another day* and push it off. But trying new things has a way of leading to bigger and better things.

What have you always wanted to try? Maybe some of your ideas seem silly, but who cares? Sign up for the tai chi lesson or go to a painting class. Meet new people on a hiking meetup or try indoor mountain climbing. Instead of alcohol, you're now the active agent in creating your own fun. Next time someone asks you what you do if you don't drink, how about giving them this answer?: *live.*

This week, you'll brainstorm a bucket list of things you want to do, have, or be in this lifetime. And to get started on things to do, here are some ideas:

- Painting or drawing
- Making music
- Playing games
- Writing short stories, poems, or articles
- Cooking new cuisines
- Scrapbooking
- Gardening
- Dancing salsa or tango
- Doing martial arts, Zumba, or CrossFit
- Fishing
- Playing tennis
- Starting a podcast
- Going to a museum or art gallery
- Starting a blog or website
- Riding a bike

- Learning to sail or windsurf
- Joining an improv group
- Stargazing
- Bird watching
- Learning a new language
- Doing macramé
- Volunteering
- Traveling

And the list goes on and on. Find something that allows you to get into flow. Mihaly Csikszentmihalyi, the leading psychologist and academic behind the concept of flow, theorizes that "people are happiest when they are in a state of flow—a state of concentration or complete absorption with the activity at hand and the situation. It is a state in which people are so involved in an activity that nothing else seems to matter. We are often happiest when we are engaged in activities that we think are important, we are passionate about, we find challenging, and we think we're good at."[1] Letting yourself play and explore inspires you, and you have no idea where it could lead.

USE JEALOUSY TO YOUR ADVANTAGE

As you explore new things, you're on the hunt for what brings you flow, excitement, and a sense of purpose. Another great tool to tap into is jealousy. While being jealous of other people often doesn't feel good, it's an incredible tool that can point you to your purpose. As a drinker, I used to be a really jealous person. I was jealous of people who had a bigger and richer circle of friends than me. I was jealous of people who traveled more than me. I was jealous of people who seemed more in love. I was jealous of people who made more money. I was jealous of people who were more fit. And most of all, I was jealous of people who wrote books, gave advice and helped people, built their livelihood around their passions, and had a freedom lifestyle.

You could say I was a petty, small person. But my jealousy was pointing to something much larger. It was a road map to guide me to the very things that I needed in my life to feel fulfilled. As writer Julia Cameron put it, "My jealousy had actually been a mask for my fear of doing something I really wanted to do but was not yet brave enough to take action forward."[2] Being jealous made it easier to stay stuck and judge other people rather than doing the work that would bring me closer to my dreams. Going alcohol-free gave me the courage and bravery to make those changes in my life. I started going out of my way to make more friends, instead of being angry at the world for not giving me more of them. I put myself out there by going to meetups and events. I discarded my attitude that thought leaders are lucky or that I deserve to make more money and started building my coaching business and platform, step by step. I devoted more quality time with my husband and shared more of my inner life with him—we've rebonded deeply since then. Instead of wishing I was more fit, I trained for a half-marathon and ran it. Instead of being bitter about all the people younger than me who had written books, I started waking up earlier and, well, writing this book.

Going after my passions and working toward my goals feels a lot better than being bitter and jealous. The jealousy is there for a reason—to help you know what you want in your life. Gretchen Rubin, bestselling author and leading happiness expert (also a nondrinker), used the overarching message of jealousy to transform her life and career. She was a lawyer and living an up-and-coming lawyer's dream, clerking for Supreme

Court Justice Sandra Day O'Connor. But she realized it wasn't her dream. When she thought about her friends from college and her network, she allowed herself to think of which ones she was jealous of. The answer? The friends who went into writing careers.[3] That's what she really wanted to do, and it wasn't long before Gretchen became a writer herself, and to date she's authored several bestselling books. I love how she was able to take a negative thought pattern, jealousy, and use it for her own self-discovery.

I want you to take a lesson from the people you feel jealous of, because those feelings will give you clarity into what you wish you were doing. Think of three people you feel jealousy toward. Maybe someone from your high school class wrote a book or got their doctorate or is a public speaker, and it drives you nuts. Or you could be jealous of a public figure. Once you determine why you're jealous of them (for example, you're jealous of a famous public speaker because you believe, deep down, that you have a message to share or way to inspire others), do an action step this week that moves you closer to that goal. Do a public speaking workshop, or join Toastmasters International. Taking a break from alcohol not only helps you feel the way you want to feel, but also helps you do the things you wish you did.

HOW TO GET MOTIVATED

As you gather your ideas this week, you'll find that they all still require work. You know you want to start writing a memoir about your unusual childhood, but you just don't *feel* like doing it. When you think of a happy, fulfilling life, I bet that the last thing you'd imagine is sitting in front of the TV eating chips. You know that in order to feel happy, you have to eat well, move your body, find your passions, create things, connect with others, and have fun. But in the moment? That TV sounds much more appealing. It can be hard to do the things we know would make us happier. Maybe we'll *feel* like it later.

Trust me, I rarely *feel* like it, at first. If I waited until I was in the mood to do something valuable, I'd be waiting a long time. When I trained for a half-marathon, I rarely ever felt like running. Yet when I did, I'd feel happy and proud of myself. It helped clear my mind and gave me some beautiful time to myself. I hardly ever *feel* like writing either. So I write first thing in the morning, before I can make excuses or procrastinate. I've learned that successful people don't wait to *feel* like doing the things that make them successful. While exercising, writing, or working on the business plan might feel uncomfortable at first, procrastinating feels a lot worse.

Motivation isn't a magical feeling that strikes from the beyond. It's the other way around. Act first, and then you'll be motivated. Find the first baby step that you can do, and then the universe will show you the next baby step. You don't have to manically do everything at once, only to burn out. Baby steps add up. Think of the smallest baby step you can do to get started on your passion. Then, as the Nike slogan goes, Just Do It. Just start the outline, just sign up for the class, just go for the run, just make the call, just write the section, just declutter the closet. You'll feel much happier afterward. And you're not merely getting the thing done. You're building your courage and confidence to go after anything you desire.

GET READY FOR THE BEST VACATIONS!

I bet you've been feeling unstoppable lately, yet when you picture going on that trip to the beach or foreign country, romantic images of wine at sunset or margaritas fill your mind. It's time to smash the biggest myth of all: alcohol makes vacations better. Letting go of the myth that alcohol is central to travel was the last and biggest myth I made peace with. I thought vacations were made for letting loose. I fundamentally believed you couldn't experience a place without experiencing the local drinking culture. If you're thinking the same, you're not alone. This is something my clients romanticize until they finally try it another way and discover how magical it is to vacation alcohol-free.

First off, let's kill some of that romanticism. You might be imagining the highlights of the future—a glass of champagne at a rooftop bar, a glass of wine at a nice restaurant. But is that how most of your drinking memories feel? I don't remember the highlights. What stuck with me are the lowlights. You've already done vacations with alcohol. Are all those happy, rosy memories? What about the time you drank too many mai tais and had to skip the snorkeling trip the next day? What about the time you stayed up late drinking with friends and had to wake up for a 5:00 a.m. flight, still burping up the alcohol? So gross. What about the time at the beach that you day drank and never even swam? What about all the times you felt so tired and exhausted after your vacation, you wish you had another vacation just to recover? Most adults drink every day on vacation. It's exhausting!

When I think of all the money and time I saved to go on vacations, today it strikes me as incongruent to visit one of the most beautiful tropical places in the world and sit around a dark bar. Or be in a capital culture of the world and vote for brewery over museum. Or waste any day feeling out of it or sluggish. Getting clear that alcohol hasn't made your vacations better and in fact added a lot of baggage is important. And when you travel alcohol-free, you're not just experiencing the world minus the baggage. If you've felt even a hint of the magic of being fully alive back at home, it increases threefold when you travel. I experience so much wonder and awe in natural beauty, majestic temples, and cultural masterpieces. I'm never looking for a bigger and better reward and fully immerse myself in what I'm experiencing.

First, start with an open mind. You've drank on vacations before. The alcohol-free way could blow your mind. Allow yourself the possibility that you'll fall in love with it, as all of my clients have. They eat at nice restaurants, laugh with their friends, and wake up the next day to watch the sunrise or go for a run. Remember the alcohol-free mantra: more not less.

I got to experience it for myself rather quickly. I traveled a lot in my first year alcohol-free. I proved to myself that every place—from the tropics to the European classics to Latin America to Asia to even big drinking cites—were much more fun without alcohol. My first trip, at thirty days alcohol-free, was a social justice immersion trip to New Orleans, with some colleagues from my previous job. I'd been to New Orleans before, and memories of the Big Easy were tinged with the pain of drinking too much. This time I went out to dinners and jazz clubs and bars, and I was struck with the peace of not having to worry about drinking too much or not getting enough sleep.

One night, I was in a hip backyard live music bar. My co-workers and I stayed there and enjoyed the live music for about four hours. When I pictured the alternative of how many drinks I would have had in a four-hour period, even if I paced myself, it would have been too many to sleep well. I would have been stressed about staying up late, knowing we had a big day the next day. Instead, I chilled, got into the vibe, and had nothing to worry about. It was a whole new way of experiencing live music, and I liked it. I woke up at 7:00 a.m., ready to appreciate another day. Hearing my coworkers complain that they hadn't slept well (and knowing exactly what the culprit was) made me feel lucky.

Then there was Hawaii, which blew me away. I didn't waste a single moment there. I woke up early to watch the sunrise. I did yoga on the beach. I swam as much as possible. I hiked. I snorkeled. I watched every sunset with awe—not trying to find an outdoor bar to get a drink to make the sunset better. Nature was good enough. I rented bikes and explored the coastline. I went on foodie adventures. It was eye-opening for me.

And one day on that trip, the universe showed me the contrast. At the beach I met a woman around my age. She seemed nice, and we chatted for a while. Then she invited me to a bar for a drink. I told her I didn't drink but would go for an alcohol-free drink. We got to a bar, and she ordered a double drink and a shot, while I nursed my nonalcoholic beer. Everything went blotto for her after that, and as we walked back to the beach, she was slurring and getting sentimental about an ex. She invited me out for her friend's birthday that evening. I declined, but we agreed to get breakfast at this great udon place the next morning.

As we parted I couldn't even imagine what kind of day she would have after that—but I could, because I'd lived it myself. Drunk at the beach by 1:00 p.m., there was nothing else for her to do that day except pass out and sleep or drink more. No swimming, no hiking, no adventures across the island. Compound that by a crazy night out, and I would have been done for the next day.

Surprise, surprise—she never showed for breakfast the next morning, and I didn't hear from her for the rest of the trip. I remember the pain of saying one thing and not living in integrity with it. I knew how disingenuous she must have felt, even if she tried to brush it off. Who had the better trip in Hawaii? The woman living it up with mai tais or the woman soaking up every moment of paradise? I've already lived that other woman's life. There is absolutely no comparison.

When you travel the world alcohol-free, you get to see it and experience it fully. Get excited about how the world will open up for you, and have fun exploring alcohol-free drinks around the world. From agua frescas to local craft sodas to calorie-free nonalcoholic Japanese beer, there's a lot out there for you.

WEEK 7 MOCKTAIL

PASSION FRUIT ZINGER

Playing with different juices, teas, fruit, and sparkling water combos is fun. Expand your tea selection and experiment with making mocktails with jasmine green tea, spiced tea, and vanilla tea.

MAKES 1 SERVING

- 120ml passion fruit juice
- 60ml vanilla tea, steeped and cooled
- Juice of half a lime
- Mint, for garnish

Put the passion fruit juice, vanilla tea, and lime juice in a shaker with ice and shake vigorously. Pour the mixture in a tall glass with ice and garnish with fresh mint.

YOUR JOURNALING HOMEWORK

I hope you're excited about all the incredible ways you get to encounter this world. I want you to make a bucket list of all the activities or experiences you want to try in your lifetime. Think of fifty out-of-the-box things you'd like to experience one day—things you want to do, have, or be. You can think of fun stuff, like zip-lining or seeing the Northern Lights (do), owning a business or a house by the sea (have), and becoming a writer or millionaire (be).

Once you have your list, what are three things you could realistically challenge yourself to do in the next ninety days?

I want you to start one today! Sign up for the French lessons. Buy the website domain. Research that trip to Japan. Take a baby step today to finish or start one of the items on your bucket list.

Step into Your Purpose

This last week together is all about going deep to answer the ultimate question: What do I want to do with my life? How do I take the dreams and goals I put on the back burner and chart a course to go after them today? And how can I use my unique gifts in service of others and step into my fullest potential?

You've decluttered your mind and now have a blank canvas to work with. It's time to fill it in with the things that matter most. The profundity of your life lies in the meaning and purpose you make of it. You are good enough, worthy enough, smart enough, and capable enough for your dreams. This journey has always been about much more than a beverage or whether or not you drink—it's about discovering the life you were meant to live. It's my favorite part of the process!

SOMEDAY GOALS

You know those someday goals from Someday Isle that feel more like wishes on the back burner? Those goals and dreams you'd love to achieve, eventually, down the line, someday, when you have more time and motivation? Maybe you didn't apply for the new job opening at your company because you're worried that you won't get the promotion. Maybe you're doing great at work but are terrified to venture out on your own and start the business you've been dreaming of. Maybe you've been thinking about going back to school for an advanced degree, but it will involve a lot of extra time and work. Or maybe you feel called to explore a new pursuit, like writing a book or starting your own nonprofit, but you have no idea where to begin.

You and only you are responsible for transforming yourself into that someday version of you. It's time to go after your someday goals, instead of allowing the inertia caused by indecision and disbelief to limit you. It's time to stop believing the lie that you're not capable. It's time to stop playing it safe. Fear almost always manifests as a logic and reasoning. It's like the comptroller of your brain, telling you all the risks and impossibilities that immediately close doors. You have to pay the bills, right? And you don't even know how to do websites. And blogging is so 2005. Plus, let's not forget the bills and the mortgage again!

When I look back, if I wanted to write, was there anything stopping me? Were the bills not going to be handled because I devoted a few hours on the side of my day job to write? Of course not. But I never even allowed myself to start, because I believed there was no money in writing, so I gave up without ever having written a word. What a waste. My realistic reasons for not chasing my dreams were a thin veil for fear. So, what's stopping you from chasing your dreams?

Let me ask you this: If money weren't an issue, how would you spend the next year? Personally, I'd travel, speak on stages, meet really cool people, write, and scale my business that inspires soul seekers to stop playing small with a beverage and tap into their fullest potential. Drinking makes it easy to keep doing the same things and have the same routine because it numbs the signal that you're not living your dream in the first place. Mix in adulthood, bills, other people's expectations, and the real problem, fear, and it's no wonder chasing our dream lives isn't the norm in our world.

This is the perfect time to do some soul-searching. I'm not asking you to quit your job tomorrow and go study Buddhism in Nepal for a year. I'm asking you to reflect and start taking small steps toward the passions that lie on your heart. It's often not reality that stops us from working on our someday goals and dreams, but fear.

You wouldn't have the dreams you have if you weren't capable of fulfilling them. Not everyone dreams about writing a book. Not everyone dreams about helping women find economic opportunity. Not everyone dreams about being an artist. You have the exact dreams you have because you have the potential to manifest them. Your dreams choose you for a reason, and it's an honor to receive them. Don't pretend you don't have what it takes, so you can play it safe. Feeling the fear and doing it anyway is what grows you to achieve the dream. You're meant to feel this way! A mantra that I love to repeat to myself is "faith over fear." You mix faith with baby steps, and doors open for you.

A UNIQUE GIFT

You are a bright light with a unique gift to share with the world. Only you can share this exact gift because no one out there has the identical perspective, experience, interests, and mentality that you do. There has never been anyone like you on this planet, and there never will be again. Your gift not only gives you meaning and value, but it serves the world. It's meant to make the world a better, happier, and more conscious place. Maybe a part of you has always known you are meant for more, and this realization terrified you. You didn't want to be singled out and magnanimous. Alcohol was a great solution to dim that light, blend in, and try to be like everyone else, by drinking over your creative force. It seemed easier to stay in your comfort zone than to dream big, play big, and dare big. We're not just scared of failure—we're also scared of success. Because when we shine bright, we're terrified of outshining others and losing belonging and acceptance. But ignore your light, and you'll feel regretful for what could have been. Your unique gift was given to you by the universe. Your fears are no match for its full support.

Do you have any ideas about what your unique gift to the world may be? Maybe it's your artistic vision or passion for changemaking. Maybe it's sharing your story to inspire others or helping others overcome the challenges you've overcome. Who knows? The world has never seen you in your full potential before. If you're not sure where to start, ask yourself what social causes pull on your heart. Can you remember the first social cause you felt strongly about? Maybe it was cleaning up your local beach or girls' empowerment. Maybe it was ending child hunger or buying more locally or ethically.

When I was in high school and college, I was passionate about women's equality. I supported women's art, wrote essays, and engaged in bold conversations about change. Unfortunately, over the years my drinking identity took away my passions for finding solutions to humanity's greatest challenges. It's hard to fight for change or innovate new solutions when you feel small and stuck. Today, I take that same yearning to make a difference by helping women achieve their greatest potential outside a beverage. The world needs you as a full-spirited, clear-headed, and passionate leader. As the saying goes, if not you, then who? If not now, then when? Your purpose aligns with serving the world. The possibilities of how you can use your drive and voice are endless.

You were never meant to dim your light and blend in. Being normal is also being mediocre, average, and boring. Wishing you were normal or different is a waste of your beautiful energy. Imagine if I hadn't spent years focusing on whether my drinking was normal. I would have freed up so much mental energy and potential, to figure out what it is I want to be and do, much sooner.

MANIFEST YOUR DREAMS

When you know you're made for more yet keep swirling in doubts and fears, it's hard to act according to your dreams. While the doubts and fears won't ever completely go away (or, more accurately, they'll evolve as you grow and uplevel), it's important to give your mind enough positive belief and emotion to counteract your doubts and fears, so you can go for it. If you 100 percent believe you can't do something, I don't know how it would be possible for your actions to prove otherwise. Imagine a baseball player at bat repeatedly telling herself, *I won't be able to hit the ball.* Why would her body do anything different? She's already preprogrammed her results through her beliefs. Your actions follow what you think—you will prove your beliefs right.

Two ways to change your thoughts and beliefs so they align with what you do want in your life are affirmations and visualization. An affirmation is a statement that's part of the process of telling yourself a new story. You could write down your affirmations, say them in front of the mirror, or repeat them like a mantra when working out (my personal fave). Remember that most of your thoughts are negative and repeat day after day. You must become intentional about what you choose to focus on. Saying or writing down affirmations is a declaration to the universe and to your subconscious about what you do want in your life. Repetition is powerful, especially if you couple it with body movement and let yourself feel excited and happy.

You can take any goal or dream you have for yourself and state it as an affirmation. Write or say it in the present tense— for example, *I'm a successful full-time entrepreneur,* or *I write a bestselling book. I'm a millionaire.* You can also use affirmations like mantras, to pep yourself up: *I deserve to live the life of my dreams. I am confident, fulfilled, and achieving. Everything I need to achieve my goals is already inside me.*

Visualization is another powerful technique to step into faith over fear. Visualizing is like meditation, only you daydream about the goals you have for yourself. You could visualize traveling the world and having a freedom lifestyle. You could visualize having your name called for a top award. You could visualize money rolling in from your business. In essence, you can trick your subconscious into believing your dreams are possible. Visualization familiarizes your dreams in your mind and places them in the realm of possibilities. Visualizing not only chips away at self-limiting beliefs, it also creates intense positive feelings. You can focus on the negative all day and feel pretty shitty as a result. Or you can visualize your dream life and feel amazing. It's up to you. This week, I'll walk you through a visualization exercise to get you started.

SPIRITUAL GROWTH

When you're open to trusting your inner wisdom and putting down the things that make you play small, you're growing yourself spiritually. My client Samantha said it succinctly: Drinking hindered her spiritual growth. Without it, she's deepened her connection with what you could call God, source, the universe, or her higher self. In many ways, the intuitive nudge to make changes in the first place is a message from divine wisdom. The very act itself is listening to the call. One of my clients told me that before we started working together, he knew he was meant to be part of a spiritual movement, but that he wouldn't be able to step into that calling until he figured out the role of alcohol in his life. Today, happily alcohol-free and using his evenings to pray and meditate, he's the embodiment of the leader he always wanted to be and building a modern spiritual movement online.

Our spiritual sides allow us to ask deep questions and find meaning and faith. For me, faith means trusting the universe and its guidance. I trust the connection in all things and that life is always unfolding for me, not to me. I see serendipity and witness synchronicities all the time. I invite in moments of silence and try to listen to the answers. The journey you're on is a journey back to your intrinsic self. You're removing the clutter, the bullshit beliefs that don't serve you, other people's expectations, and learning to stand in your power.

The woman I thought needed a drink to have fun is long dead, because she was a construction of the society around me. She fed off the fears society told me to have—that I'm shy, awkward, and insignificant—and in order to guard herself from these fears, she found a security blanket in alcohol. But deep down, underneath those limiting thoughts and fears, was a truer version of me. The one connected to my higher self and my purpose.

Challenging yourself not to drink helps you understand and learn from your emotions and become aware of your thoughts. You learn how to observe yourself and know yourself. When you know that any uncomfortable feeling is temporary and fleeting and let yourself truly feel it instead of numbing it, you grow your resiliency and emotional strength. You evolve. In fact, you develop more resiliency, strength, and flexibility than someone who never had to deal with this at all. It's proven in the new neural pathways you've built in your brain and the ones you've pruned because they don't serve you. This so-called problem has been in your life for a purpose: so it could help grow you into an expanded version of yourself. You are here to transcend your challenges and limitations, to grow and uncover your radiance and truth.

STEP INTO YOUR PURPOSE

Martha Beck, author of *Finding Your Own North Star*, shares a journal exercise to help you uncover your greater purpose. Imagine it's ten years from now, and you're on the cover of your favorite magazine.[1] They're highlighting you because of your incredible contribution to humanity and to celebrate your success. What are you being honored for? What have you done that serves others and gives you meaning? What is your legacy?

Asking yourself big questions like this helps you tap into a deeper part of your being. In our society, it's abnormal to ask ourselves how to live in alignment with our deeper passions, unique expression, and big dreams. Maybe you used to dream big when you were younger, but adulthood drove you to settle into the pressures of reality and emulate society's expectations or other people's dreams. It's easy to work at a company and absorb everyone else's goal of moving up the ladder, without asking yourself if that's what you want. We're taught to work hard to make our parents proud and get a certain degree or job title, without asking if that's what will fulfill us. My good friend Chelsea worked for years to become a doctor, only to realize the medical field was making her miserable. It took a lot of courage to go deep within herself and find what she really wanted to do. Today, she's a career coach, travels the world, and is supremely happy.

I know it's easy to write this all off and doubt you could do what you love and make a living off of it. Martha Beck wrote that "When you're doing what you're meant to do, you benefit the world in a unique and irreplaceable way. This brings money, friendship, true love, inner peace, and everything else worth having; it sounds facile, but it's really true."[2] You never know what will happen if you pursue your passions, even with the tiniest baby steps. Action begets opportunities. And the regret you'll feel for playing it safe and unfulfilled will weigh on you much more than the fear of taking a chance.

Problems come into your life for a reason. Usually they're intended to wake you up from the ways you've settled and veered off the path of your true purpose. Having a complicated relationship with alcohol is a gift because through it, you're waking up to your greatness and potential. Anything is possible for you, and your dreams chose you for a reason. You're the exact person who was meant to bring them about and heal the world through your unique gifts. We're waiting for you!

●　●　●

──── YOUR JOURNALING HOMEWORK ────

Find a quiet place in your house and set the mood. Put on some meditation music and do four rounds of box breathing (in for the count of four, hold for the count of four, exhale for the count of four, and hold at the bottom for the count of four). In your journal, allow yourself to dream your ideal life within the following categories:

- Legacy and mission/career
- Romantic relationship
- Family, friends, and network
- Health and wellness
- Financial wealth
- Travel and lifestyle

Write five sentences (in the present tense) of what you'd love to have in each category in your dream life. For example, for romantic relationship I could write: I have a soulmate marriage. In health and wellness, I could write: I'm an avid cyclist. In travel, I write: I spend months crisscrossing Europe. For each category, take a few moments to imagine your sentences coming true. Picture yourself in that Roman café, having an espresso and biscotti in front of the Pantheon. See yourself waking up with the sunrise to go cycling across the countryside in the early morning light. Visualize yourself with a devoted and loving partner. Picture the business, the money, the impact, the magnitude of your desires fully manifesting for you. Really use your imagination.

If you uncovered new goals and life dreams for yourself, that's amazing. Use these visions as new affirmations in your journaling and get started on the smallest baby step today.

Celebrate!

You did it! You just spent the past eight weeks completely reevaluating your life, letting go of what no longer fits who you want to become, and becoming that person instead. This is huge, and I'm proud of you. Whether you went all eight-weeks sans alcohol or had a few slips doesn't matter. What matters is the way you've grown and shown up for yourself. You know yourself much better now, and I'm grateful the universe gave us a chance to connect.

I have an important assignment for you right now: I want you to celebrate! You looked at a not-so-glamorous habit with vulnerability and courage. You asked tough questions. You answered from your heart. You learned. You grew. You expanded. So get up from your chair, put on your favorite feel-good song, and dance for at least two minutes straight, with joy and excitement for accomplishing the work you've done.

Then, celebrate yourself with a cool reward. Alcohol and celebration have been tied together by society for too long, so sever that tie by finding something that makes you feel alive. Buy that weekend yoga retreat you've been wanting to go on for years, or plan that camping weekend with your buddies. Make reservations at the fanciest restaurant in town. Get a massage or go to an amusement park. Whatever it is, find something you truly deserve to treat yourself with. And grab your phone, take another selfie, and compare it to the one you took eight weeks ago. Notice a difference? I bet you do.

WHAT NOW?

Once you're done honoring yourself for your massive accomplishment, you might be wondering what comes next on your journey. You could consciously choose to drink, or you could extend your break. It's up to you.

If your next step forward comes with slips back into drinking, use this as a learning opportunity. You can't unknow the information you've read in this book, and your new perspective can help you determine what feels good in your life and what doesn't. If you drink and notice more negative emotions or rough sleep that you don't want to invite into your life, use that as a sign to take another break.

My goal with this book is to help you grow and develop into a more self-loving, resilient, and capable version of you. One aligned to your deeper values and bigger dreams. It's not really about sobriety, per se—it's about designing a life you love so much that drinking loses its allure. If drinking was a way of playing small and hiding from your life, why ever play small again? Life is too magical, and you are too bright a star to dull.

Whatever you decide, make growth a new nonnegotiable in your life and keep expanding your potential. If you decide to extend your break (woo-hoo!), pick a number of months, and go for it! You'll never regret it. When the future version of you looks back at today, she'll be so proud. She's cheering you on!

BE AN ALCOHOL-FREE REBEL

Sometimes I like to think of a future where alcohol completely goes by the wayside. A hundred years from now, as we continue to advance as a society, we're not going to keep ingesting a toxin that lowers our lifespan, just to get a buzz. Alcohol will be considered a crude chemical that caused cancer, and there will probably be other popular, mood-enhancing drinks available. Today's younger generations are way more likely to be alcohol-free, and this shift will change our culture.[1] If you doubt me and my predictions, by claiming that alcohol has been around since the dawn of civilized humanity, consider how our culture has shifted away from cigarette smoking being a socially acceptable activity. One day, alcohol will lose its favor the way cigarette smoking did, and you must ask yourself: Do I want to be in the front of that bell curve as an early adopter, in the middle, or one of the last stragglers?

Alcohol is the new cigarette. It's the contradiction of our conscious times to do everything to be healthy but not consider excluding alcohol, and then make anyone who doesn't drink feel like something is wrong with them. The illusion that drinking makes us feel cool, sophisticated, romantic, or adventurous is just that—an illusion. Stand up to it, stand up to conditioning, stand up to the messages that say you're not enough on your own, and stand up to the idea that you have to drink to fit in.

If being alcohol-free over the past eight weeks allowed you to express yourself and dream bigger, it's worth being a radical. Tap into your inner activism and rebelliousness as you navigate the world as a nondrinker.

Welcome to the rebel club.

ACKNOWLEDGMENTS

It's hard to believe that this dream that I've fantasized about since I was a little girl has come true. First, I want to thank her—that little girl gave me the vision a long time ago that this was possible.

Thank you to everyone who helped bring this book to life. Wendy Sherman, for championing and believing in its potential. Callie Deitrick, for recognizing its value. Richelle Fredson, for mining the diamond out of the rough. Thanks to everyone on the Harper Horizon team who helped me so much. Special thanks to Amanda Bauch, Andrea Fleck-Nisbet, and John Andrade for your invaluable expertise, editing, and support. Thank you to Patti Zorr, Kathleen Carter, and Rob Eager for helping me get it into the hands of readers.

Thank you to my team at Euphoric—I couldn't do what I do without you! Barbara, you are my lifeblood. Alison and Steve, you make our content sound amazing. Danielle, you've helped us grow so much.

To my entrepreneur friends and alcohol-free sisters for inspiring me. Danielle Baldino, you helped me beyond words to start this entrepreneurial journey. My sister circle, you're there for me every single week with encouragement and love—thank you! Cailen Ascher and Melyssa Griffin, you've guided me toward an expansive, abundant life, and I'm so thankful for you. Annie Grace, thank you for starting a movement and sharing the keys to the castle.

ACKNOWLEDGMENTS

To my clients and students, you inspire me! Thank you for asking me to come alongside you to help you realize your beautiful gifts. What a privilege!

To my online mentors, who have changed my world and uplift me to believe in my biggest dreams: Tony Robbins, you empower me to live a beautiful, impactful life. Big thank you to Rachel Hollis, Brendon Burchard, Denise Duffield-Thomas, Marie Forleo, Dean Graziosi, and Jenna Kutcher.

To the bravery my parents showed to leave the only home they ever knew, with no more than a suitcase of clothes and the hope that life could be better. Their hard work and love have given me everything I needed to succeed. *Serdecznie dziekuje.* Katie, you've been my rock my whole life—thank you for your love and support.

Lastly, to Robert. Thank you for being the most loving, supportive, believing husband I could ever ask for. You saw the possibilities, and you got on the train with me. I love you.

And one final thank you to Huxley, my fluffy Samoyed, for all the sweet cuddles and kisses he gave me throughout.

NOTES

INTRODUCTION

1. National Health Service (United Kingdom), "Alcohol Units, Alcohol Support," https://www.nhs.uk/live-well/alcohol-support/calculating-alcohol-units/.

2. Centers for Disease Control and Prevention (CDC), "Dietary Guidelines for Alcohol," https://www.cdc.gov/alcohol/fact-sheets/moderate-drinking.htm.

3. Centers for Disease Control and Prevention (CDC), "Alcohol Use and Your Health," https://www.cdc.gov/alcohol/fact-sheets/alcohol-use.htm.

4. Substance Abuse and Mental Health Services Administration, "Key Substance Use and Mental Health Indicators in the United States: Results from the 2019 National Survey on Drug Use and Health," September 2020, publication ID PEP20-07-01-001, https://store.samhsa.gov/product/key-substance-use-and-mental-health-indicators-in-the-united-states-results-from-the-2019-national-survey-on-Drug-Use-and-Health/PEP20-07-01-001?referer=from_search_result.

5. Centers for Disease Control and Prevention (CDC), "Alcohol and Public Health: Frequently Asked Questions," https://www.cdc.gov/alcohol/faqs.htm#.

6. Vanessa Romo and Allison Aubrey, "U.S. Alcohol-Related Deaths Have Doubled, Study Says," January 8, 2020, NPR, https://www.npr.org/2020/01/08/794772148/alcohol-related-deaths-have-doubled-study-says.

7. Anne Sampson, "The Low Down: As Consumers Focus on Healthful Trends, Beverage Companies Are Responding with Low Calorie, Low Sugar, and Low (Even No) Alcohol Options," November 13, 2019, Spirited, https://www.spiritedbiz.com/the-low-down-as-consumers-focus-on-healthful-trends-beverage-companies-are-responding-with-low-calorie-low-sugar-and-low-even-no-alcohol-options/.

8. One Year No Beer (website), accessed May 16, 2021, https://www.oneyearnobeer.com/90-day-challenge/.

9. Kendra Cherry, "What Is Cognitive Dissonance?" Verywell Mind, July 2, 2020, https://www.verywellmind.com/what-is-cognitive-dissonance-2795012.

CHAPTER 2

1. William Porter, Alcohol Explained, blog and podcasts, 2018, https://www.alcoholexplained.com/.

2. Danielle Pacheco, "Alcohol and Sleep," Sleep Foundation, September 4, 2020, https://www.sleepfoundation.org/articles/how-alcohol-affects-quality-and-quantity-sleep.

3. Irshaad O. Ebrahim et al., "Alcohol and Sleep I: Effects on Normal Sleep," *Alcoholism: Clinical and Experimental Research* 37, no .4 (April 2013): 539–49, https://doi.org/10.1111/acer.12006.

4. Timothy Roehrs and Thomas Roth, "Sleep, Sleepiness, and Alcohol Use," National Institute on Alcohol Abuse and Alcoholism, https://pubs.niaaa.nih.gov/publications/arh25-2/101-109.htm.

5. Robert L. Spencer and Kent E. Hutchison, "Alcohol, Aging, and the Stress Response," National Institute on Alcohol Abuse and Alcoholism, https://pubs.niaaa.nih.gov/publications/arh23-4/272-283.pdf.

6. Spencer and Hutchison.

7. Ebrahim et al., "Alcohol and Sleep I."

8. Andrea Rock, *The Mind at Night: The New Science of How and Why We Dream* (New York: Basic Books, 2004).

9. Shingo Kitamura et al., "Estimating Individual Optimal Sleep Duration and Potential Sleep Debt," *Scientific Reports* 6 (October 24, 2016): 35812, https://doi.org/10.1038/srep35812.

10. Kate Taylor, "Millennials Are Dragging Down Beer Sales—but Gen Z Marks a 'Turning Point' That Will Cause an Even Bigger Problem for the Industry," February 21, 2018, *Insider*, https://www.businessinsider.com/millennials-gen-z-drag-down-beer-sales-2018-2?r=UK.

11. Joanna Piacenza, "People Are Drinking Less, but Don't Blame Millennials," August 8, 2018, Morning Consult, https://morningconsult.com/2019/08/08/people-are-drinking-less-but-dont-blame-millennials/.

NOTES

CHAPTER 3

1. Karolina Rzadkowolska, "18: One Year No Beer with Andy Ramage," June 19, 2019, in *Euphoric The Podcast* (podcast), 1:11:55, https://www.euphoricaf.com/the-podcast/andy-ramage.

2. Lindsay Dodge, "Working Out with a Hangover Is a Terrible Idea According to Fitness Experts—Here's Why," June 13, 2018, *Insider*, https://www.insider.com/why-you-shouldnt-work-out-with-a-hangover-2018-6.

3. Dodge.

4. Michael Greger, "How Many Servings of Fruits and Vegetables to Improve Mood?," September 4, 2018, Nutrition Facts, https://nutritionfacts.org/2018/09/04/how-many-servings-of-fruits-and-vegetables-to-improve-mood/.

5. Charles Duhigg, *The Power of Habit: Why We Do What We Do in Life and Business* (New York: Random House, 2014).

CHAPTER 4

1. Sarah Cains et al., "Agrp Neuron Activity Is Required for Alcohol-Induced Overeating," *Nature Communications* 8, no. 14014 (January 10, 2017), https://www.nature.com/articles/ncomms14014.

2. Gina Firth and Luis G. Manzo, "How Alcohol Affects You," Student Health Services, University of California at San Diego website, accessed May 26, 2021, https://studenthealth.ucsd.edu/resources/health-topics/alcohol-drugs/nutrition-endurance.html.

3. Scott Q. Siler, Richard A. Neese, and Marc K. Hellerstein, "De Novo Lipogenesis, Lipid Kinetics, and Whole-Body Lipid Balances in Humans after Acute Alcohol Consumption," *The American Journal of Clinical Nutrition* 70, no 5. (November 1999): 928–36, https://doi.org/10.1093/ajcn/70.5.928.

4. Firth and Manzo, "How Alcohol Affects You."

CHAPTER 5

1. Rene Wisely, "Doctors Are Seeing More Alcoholic Liver Disease among Young Adults," January 22, 2019, HealthBlog, University of Michigan

Health, https://healthblog.uofmhealth.org/digestive-health/doctors-are-seeing-more-alcoholic-liver-disease-young-adults#.

2. Gautam Mehta et al., "Short-Term Abstinence from Alcohol and Changes in Cardiovascular Risk Factors, Liver Function Tests and Cancer-Related Growth Factors: A Prospective Observational Study," *BMJ Open* 8, no. 5 (May 5, 2018):e020673, https://doi.org/10.1136/bmjopen-2017-020673.

3. Randy Dotinga, "Study Ties Alcohol Abuse to Increased Heart Risks," WebMD, January 2, 2017, https://www.webmd.com/mental-health/addiction/news/20170102/study-ties-alcohol-abuse-to-increased-heart-risks.

4. Michael Greger, "Is It Better to Drink a Little Alcohol than None at All?," (video), 5:26, April 4, 2018, NutritionFacts, https://nutritionfacts.org/video/is-it-better-to-drink-little-alcohol-than-none-at-all/.

5. Michael Greger, "The Best Source of Resveratrol," (video), 3:56, April 2, 2018, https://nutritionfacts.org/video/the-best-source-of-resveratrol/.

6. Amy Z. Fan et al., "Drinking Pattern and Blood Pressure among Non-Hypertensive Current Drinkers: Findings from 1999–2004 National Health and Nutrition Examination Survey," *Clinical Epidemiology* 5, no. 1 (January 29, 2013): 21–27, https://doi.org/10.2147/CLEP.S12152.

7. Robert Preidt, "Many Don't Know How to Handle High Cholesterol," April 11, 2017, *HealthDay News*, https://www.webmd.com/cholesterol-management/news/20170411/many-americans-dont-know-how-to-handle-high-cholesterol.

8. Centers for Disease Control and Prevention, "Facts about Hypertension," last reviewed September 8, 2020, https://www.cdc.gov/bloodpressure/facts.htm.

9. Mehta et al., "Short-Term Abstinence from Alcohol."

10. Sergey Kalinin et al., "Transcriptome Analysis of Alcohol-Treated Microglia Reveals Downregulation of Beta Amyloid Phagocytosis," *Journal of Neuroinflammation* 15, no. 141 (May 14, 2018), https://doi.org/10.1186s12974-018-1184-7.

11. Anya Topiwala, at al., "No Safe Level of Alcohol Consumption for Brain Health: Observational Cohort Study of 25,378 UK Biobank Participants," ResearchGate, May 2021, https://doi.org/10.1101/2021.05.10.21256931.

12. Marc Lewis, *The Biology of Desire: Why Addiction Is Not a Disease* (New York: PublicAffairs Books, 2015).

13. Stacy Simon, "American Cancer Society Updates Guideline for Diet and Physical Activity," June 9, 2020, American Cancer Society, https://www .cancer.org/latest-news/american-cancer-society-updates-guideline-for -diet-and-physical-activity.html.

14. Noelle K. LoConte et al., "Alcohol and Cancer: A Statement of the American Society of Clinical Oncology," *Journal of Clinical Oncology* 36, no. 1 (January 1, 2018): 83–93, https://doi.org/10.1200/JCO.2017.76.1155.

15. Kevin D. Shield, Isabelle Soerjomataram, and Jürgen Rehm, "Alcohol Use and Breast Cancer: A Critical Review," *Alcoholism: Clinical and Experimental Research* 40, no. 6 (June 2016): 1166–81, https://doi.org/10.1111/acer .13071.

16. Ananya Mandal, "Bottle of Wine Equivalent to Smoking 10 Cigarettes," March 29, 2019, News Medical, https://www.news-medical.net/news /20190329/Bottle-of-wine-equivalent-to-smoking-10-cigarettes.aspx.

17. Mehta et al., "Short-Term Abstinence from Alcohol."

18. GBD 2016 Alcohol Collaborators, "Alcohol Use and Burden for 195 Countries and Territories, 1990–2016: A Systematic Analysis for the Global Burden of Disease Study 2016," *Lancet* 392 (August 23, 2018): 1015–35, https://doi.org/10.1016/S0140-6736(18)31310-2.

19. World Health Organization Regional Office for Europe, "There Is No Safe Level of Alcohol, New Study Confirms," September 13, 2018, https://www.euro.who.int/en/health-topics/disease-prevention /alcohol-use/news/news/2018/09/there-is-no-safe-level-of-alcohol, -new-study-confirms#:~:text=There%20is%20no%20safe%20level%20 of%20alcohol%2C%20new%20study%20confirms,-AddThis%20 Sharing%20Buttons&text=The%20international%20medical%20 journal%20The,to%20loss%20of%20healthy%20life.

20. Holly Whitaker, *Quit Like a Woman: The Radical Choice to Not Drink in a Culture Obsessed with Alcohol* (London: Bloomsbury Publishing, 2020).

21. Gaetano Di Chiara, "Alcohol and Dopamine," *Alcohol Health and Research World* 21, no. 2 (1997): 108 – 14, https://www.ncbi.nlm.nih.gov/pmc /articles/PMC6826820/.

22. https://www.mentalhealth.org.uk/a-to-z/a/alcohol-and-mental-health #:~:text=One%20of%20the%20main%20problems,a%20key%20chemical %20in%20depression.

23. William Porter, *Alcohol Explained* (blog and podcast), 2018, https:// www.alcoholexplained.com/.

24. Andrew Holmes et al., "Chronic Alcohol Remodels Prefrontal Neurons and Disrupts NMDAR-Mediated Fear Extinction Encoding," *Nature Neuroscience* 15 (October 2012): 1359–61, https://doi.org/10.1038/nn.3204.

25. *Vogue*, "How to Combat the Effects of Alcohol on Skin, According to an Expert," January 15, 2020, https://www.vogue.com/article/alcohol-skin-damage-effects.

26. Ann Brenoff, "The Amount of Money You Spend on Drinking May Blow Your Mind," April 27, 2018, HuffPost, https://www.huffpost.com/entry/money-spent-on-drinking_n_5adf49d9e4b07be4d4c54401.

CHAPTER 6

1. Neringa Antanaityte, "Mind Matters: How to Effortlessly Have More Positive Thoughts," TLEX, https://tlexinstitute.com/how-to-effortlessly-have-more-positive-thoughts/.

2. As adapted from Annie Grace, *This Naked Mind: Control Alcohol, Find Freedom, Discover Happiness, & Change Your Life* (Avery, 2018).

CHAPTER 7

1. Brené Brown, *The Gifts of Imperfection* (Center City, MN.: Hazelden Publishing, 2010), p. 9.

CHAPTER 10

1. Julia Cameron, *The Artist's Way: 25th Anniversary Edition* (New York: Penguin, 2016).

CHAPTER 11

1. Johann Hari, *Lost Connections: Uncovering the Real Causes of Depression—and the Unexpected Solutions* (New York: Bloomsbury, 2018).

NOTES

CHAPTER 13

1. https://fs.blog/2019/05/gates-law/.

2. Theodore Roosevelt, "Citizenship in a Republic," Theodore Roosevelt Center at Dickinson State University, accessed May 16, 2021, https://www.theodorerooseveltcenter.org/Learn-About-TR/TR-Encyclopedia/Culture-and-Society/Man-in-the-Arena.aspx. Roosevelt gave this speech, commonly known as "The Man in the Arena," at the Sorbonne in Paris on April 23, 1910.

PART III

1. Hayley Phelan, "What's All This About Journaling," *The New York Times*, October 25, 2018, https://www.nytimes.com/2018/10/25/style/journaling-benefits.html.

2. Courtney E. Ackerman, "83 Benefits of Journaling for Depression, Anxiety, and Stress," Positive Psychology, May 19, 2021, https://positivepsychology.com/benefits-of-journaling/.

3. Joan Didion, "Joan Didion Survives *The Year of Magical Thinking*," interview by Susan Stamberg, National Public Radio, September 30, 2005, https://www.npr.org/transcripts/4866010.

WEEK 1

1. Steven Pressfield, *The War of Art: Winning the Inner Creative Battle* (London: Orion Publishing, 2003).

2. "Beat Your Cravings: 8 Effective Techniques," Mayo Clinic, accessed May 26, 2021, https://diet.mayoclinic.org/diet/eat/beat-your-cravings?xid=nl_MayoClinicDiet_20171109.

3. Ralph Ryback, "The Science of Accomplishing Your Goals," *Psychology Today*, October 3, 2016, https://www.psychologytoday.com/us/blog/the-truisms-wellness/201610/the-science-accomplishing-your-goals.

WEEK 2

1. Duhigg, *The Power of Habit*.

2. Sarah Hardey et al., "5 Most Addictive Drugs," February 22, 2021, American Addiction Centers, https://americanaddictioncenters.org/adult-addiction-treatment-programs/most-addictive.

3. Kelley Manley, "The Year of Drinking Dangerously," December 3, 2020, *Elle,* https://www.elle.com/culture/a34823556/quarantine-drinking-dangerously-2020/.

4. Jessica Fu, "Less than Half of Americans Know That Alcohol Is a Carcinogen. Big Booze Wants to Keep It That Way," December 1, 2020, The Counter, https://thecounter.org/public-health-groups-alcohol-label-warnings-carcinogen-cancer-link-awareness-prop-65/.

WEEK 4

1. Aimee Groth, "You're the Average of the Five People You Spend the Most Time With," *Business Insider,* July 24, 2012, https://www.businessinsider.com/jim-rohn-youre-the-average-of-the-five-people-you-spend-the-most-time-with-2012-7.

WEEK 5

1. Rachael E. Jack, Oliver G.B. Garrod, and Philippe G. Schyns, "Dynamic Facial Expressions of Emotion Transmit an Evolving Hierarchy of Signals over Time," *Current Biology,* January 2, 2014, https://doi.org/10.1016/j.cub.2013.11.064.

2. Neringa Antanaityte, "Mind Matters: How to Effortlessly Have More Positive Thoughts," TLEX, https://tlexinstitute.com/how-to-effortlessly-have-more-positive-thoughts/.

3. Daniel G. Amen, *Change Your Brain, Change Your Life: The Breakthrough Program for Conquering Anxiety, Depression, Anger, and Obsessiveness* (London: Piatkus Books, 2016).

4. Peter Mallouk and Tony Robbins, *The Path: Accelerating Your Journey to Financial Freedom* (London: Simon & Schuster UK, 2020).

5. Glenn N. Levine el al., "Meditation and Cardiovascular Risk Reduction: A Scientific Statement from the American Heart Association," *Journal of the American Heart Association* 6, no. 10 (September 2017), https://doi.org/10.1161/JAHA.117.002218.

NOTES

WEEK 6

1. Team Tony, "Discover the 6 Human Needs," Tony Robbins (website), accessed May 26, 2021, https://www.tonyrobbins.com/mind-meaning/do-you-need-to-feel-significant/.

2. Team Tony, "Discover the 6 Human Needs."

WEEK 7

1. Mihaly Csikszentmihalyi, *Flow: The Psychology of Optimal Experience* (New York: Harper and Row, 1990), p. 15.

2. Cameron, *The Artist's Way.*

3. Gretchen Rubin, *Better Than Before: What I Learned about Making and Breaking Habits* (New York: Broadway Books, 2015).

WEEK 8

1. Martha Beck, *Finding Your Own North Star: How to Claim the Life You Were Meant to Live* (London: Piatkus, 2004).

2. Beck.

CONCLUSION

1. Bronwyn Williams, "Teetotalism—Why Generation Z Is Choosing Good, Clean Fun," Flux, accessed May 26, 2021, https://www.fluxtrends.com/teetotalism-why-generation-z-is-choosing-good-clean-fun/.

INDEX

INDEX

Karolina Rzadkowolska is a certified alcohol-free life coach who helps powerful women make alcohol insignificant in their lives. She's worked with thousands of clients through her online courses and coaching to change their drinking habits and unleash a new level of health, happiness, and potential to go after their biggest dreams.

She's the host of *Euphoric the Podcast* and founder of Euphoric Alcohol-Free, and her work has been featured by the Huffington Post, Authority Magazine, Greatist, and Elite Daily. Karolina's passionate about helping you discover what really makes you happy outside of a beverage and design a life you love. She'd love to hear from you at www.euphoricaf.com.

She's obsessed with personal growth, loves to travel, and lives in San Diego with her husband and fluffy Samoyed.

Instagram @euphoric.af
www.euphoricaf.com